the Fit Back

Pain Relief and Prevention

FITNESS, HEALTH & NUTRITION

the Fit Back

Pain Relief and Prevention

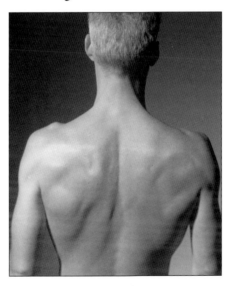

TIME® LIFE

by the Editors of Time-Life Books

CONSULTANTS FOR THIS BOOK

Deborah Caplan, a Registered Physical Therapist, specializes in back care and the Alexander Technique. A founder member of the American Center for the Alexander Technique, she is on the senior faculty of its teacher training programme.

Michael C. Neuwirth, M.D., an orthopaedic surgeon, is Chief of Scoliosis Service at the Orthopaedic Institute of the Hospital for Joint Diseases in New York.

Luanne Sforza, a Registered Physical Therapist, is Director of Physical Therapy at the Sports Training Institute in New York City; she developed the institute's Healthy Back Program.

Elaine Stillermais is a licensed massage therapist and an instructor at the Swedish Institute of Massage in New York City.

Judith C. Trobe, a Registered Physical Therapist, is a certified instructor of the Alexander Technique and frequently lectures on back care.

John White, Ph.D., is Reader in Human Performance and Health Studies at the University of Ulster at Jordanstown, Northern Ireland, with responsibilities for undergraduate teaching and postgraduate research in exercise and health studies.

NUTRITIONAL CONSULTANTS

Ann Grandjean, Ed. D., is chief nutrition consultant to the U.S. Olympic Committee and an instructor in the Sports Medicine Program, University of Nebraska Medical Center.

Myron Winick, M.D., is Professor of Nutrition at Columbia University College of Physicians and Surgeons, New York.

This edition published in 2004
by the Caxton Publishing Group
20 Bloomsbury Street, London WC1B 3JH

Under license from Time-Life Books BV.

Cover Design: Open Door Limited, Rutland UK

Title: The Fit Back

ISBN: 1 84447 162 4

This book is not intended as a substitute for the advice of a physician. Readers who have or suspect they may have specific medical problems, especially those involving muscles and joints, should consult a physician before beginning any programme of strenuous physical exercise.

CONTENTS

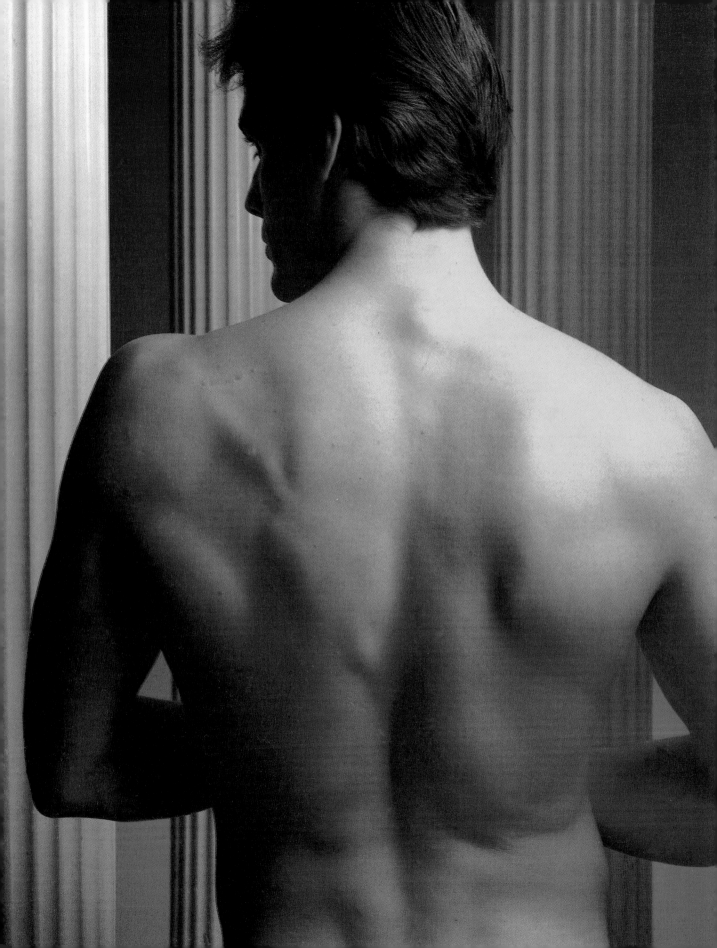

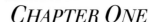

CHAPTER ONE

How Your Back Works

Its strengths and weaknesses, why backs ache and the dramatic benefits of exercise

A fit back is strong and resilient, capable of absorbing a multitude of shocks every day and of supporting loads far greater than your body weight. In well-trained athletes, a single disc in the lower back has been shown to bear loads in excess of 1,000 kilograms. Yet eight out of 10 people, including those who are generally fit, experience some type of back pain during their lives. Back problems rank second only to the common cold as the most frequent cause of sick leave in the United Kingdom and Europe, where the cost of back treatment runs into millions of pounds each year.

Much of this suffering and expense is avoidable. The great majority of all backaches stem from muscular problems that can either be prevented or alleviated with improvements in posture and exercise and other lifestyle habits. Indeed, exercising regularly is the most important step that you can take to protect your back. This chapter explains back mechanics and guides you towards effective ways in which to ease a troubled back or keep a fit back at its best.

Why should you be concerned about your back?

Just as a bad back can interfere with everyday activities, a fit back can assist you in leading an active and healthy life. The human spine — extending from the base of the skull to the tip of the coccyx — is one of the most complex and vital parts of the body. Rather than a single long bone, the spine consists of an intricate network of interlocking bones called vertebrae, fluid-filled cushioning discs, connecting ligaments, important nerves, and numerous small and large muscles that support the back (*see illustration, opposite*). This unique structure is integrally involved in almost every single movement that you make, from picking up the telephone to walking.

Although the spine is designed to accommodate everyday movement as well as the demands of exercise, it has potential weaknesses that age and repeated patterns of misuse — inactivity, poor posture habits, improper lifting, sitting in badly designed chairs — can accentuate. If your back is weak, a movement as minor as a sneeze can trigger back muscle spasms. It is therefore both sensible and prudent to care for your back before problems arise.

What causes back pain?

To some degree, all back trouble stems from degeneration. As you age, the cushioning discs separating the vertebrae of your back begin to lose some of their elasticity and moisture, and they therefore shrink. This can lead to a variety of conditions ranging from simple muscle pain to more damaging problems such as a herniated disc. Although more than 100 causes of back pain have been identified, the majority of cases are the result of injured muscles and ligaments. One large-scale university study discovered that 83 per cent of backaches could be attributed to weak or tense muscles.

Contrary to popular belief, backs do not just "give out". An accumulation of problems, including wear and tear on poorly toned muscles, bad posture, obesity and stress, are predisposing factors. A simple move, such as bending to pick up groceries, can aggravate already weakened muscles, and it may lead to a protective but painful mechanism: the back muscles go into spasm — sustained involuntary muscular contractions — to guard you from further damage. By immobilizing the back, the spasm forces you to take the best course of action and lie down. This position not only places the least amount of stress on your back, but it also allows inflamed tissue to repair itself.

Back pain varies in intensity from nagging to excruciating. The degree of pain is sometimes a good indication of the type of injury or illness, but it is sometimes misleading. Certain diseases and serious illnesses can produce low levels of back pain, while muscle spasms, which usually clear up within days, can trigger agonizing pain.

If back pain is accompanied by any change in bowel or bladder habits, decreased sexual function or numbness in the genital area, you should contact your doctor immediately. These symptoms can indicate

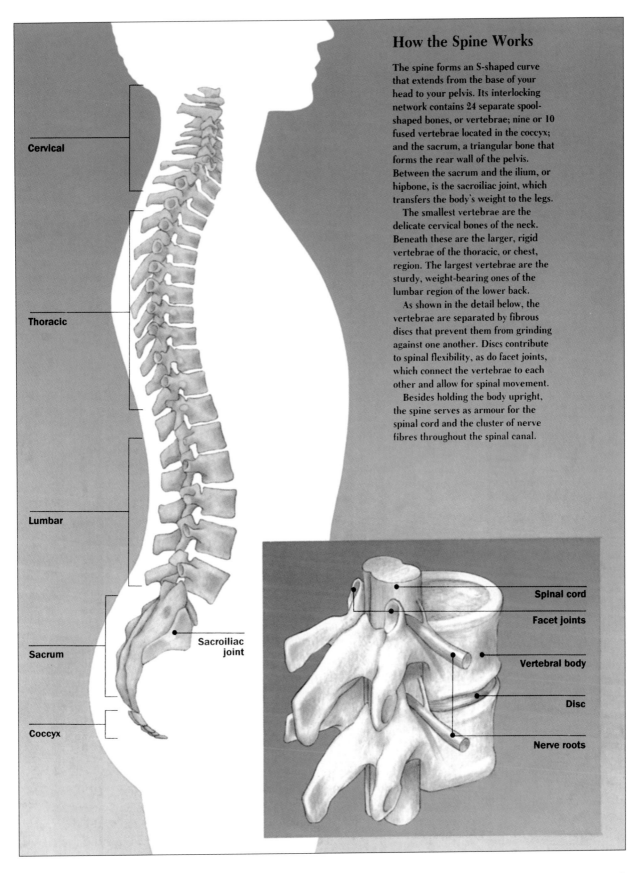

How the Spine Works

The spine forms an S-shaped curve that extends from the base of your head to your pelvis. Its interlocking network contains 24 separate spool-shaped bones, or vertebrae; nine or 10 fused vertebrae located in the coccyx; and the sacrum, a triangular bone that forms the rear wall of the pelvis. Between the sacrum and the ilium, or hipbone, is the sacroiliac joint, which transfers the body's weight to the legs.

The smallest vertebrae are the delicate cervical bones of the neck. Beneath these are the larger, rigid vertebrae of the thoracic, or chest, region. The largest vertebrae are the sturdy, weight-bearing ones of the lumbar region of the lower back.

As shown in the detail below, the vertebrae are separated by fibrous discs that prevent them from grinding against one another. Discs contribute to spinal flexibility, as do facet joints, which connect the vertebrae to each other and allow for spinal movement.

Besides holding the body upright, the spine serves as armour for the spinal cord and the cluster of nerve fibres throughout the spinal canal.

Cervical

Thoracic

Lumbar

Sacrum

Sacroiliac joint

Coccyx

Spinal cord

Facet joints

Vertebral body

Disc

Nerve roots

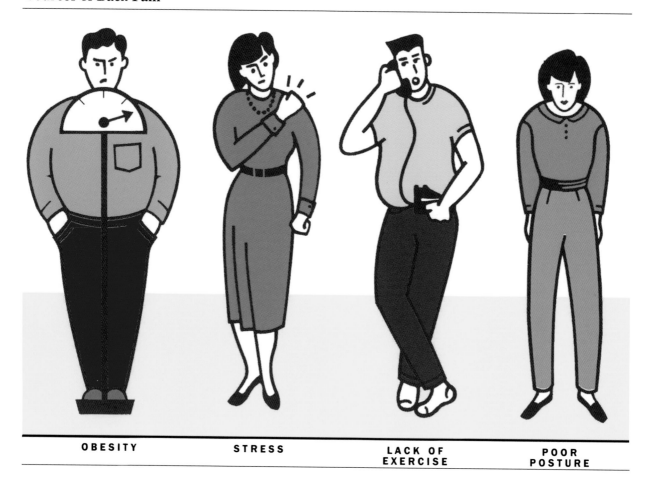

OBESITY   **STRESS**   **LACK OF EXERCISE**   **POOR POSTURE**

Each of the four factors illustrated above contributes to the likelihood of your suffering back pain. Both obesity and poor posture throw the back out of alignment, straining muscles and ligaments. Stress, the factor over which you may have the least control, can contribute to muscle tension, which increases the risk of injury and can lead to muscle spasm. A sedentary lifestyle is doubly troublesome: weak muscles fail to support the spine properly, and too much sitting causes muscular strain.

a nerve disorder that necessitates emergency surgery. Back pain accompanied by vomiting or fever or any back pain in a child should get prompt medical attention. Also, any back pain, numbness or tingling that radiates down your arm or leg, while not an emergency, should be evaluated immediately. Otherwise, experts agree that a doctor need not be contacted unless pain persists after two or three days of bed rest and aspirin or another analgesic.

Who suffers from back pain?

Although back pain can affect anyone, it is more likely to occur if you are between the ages of 30 and 55. In the United States, the average age of patients who undergo lumbar-disc surgery is 42. Because older women are more prone to osteoporosis, the bone-weakening disease, they face greater risks than older men.

Backaches afflict workers at all levels in all occupations, and those with the least physically demanding jobs may be just as vulnerable as those whose jobs are strenuous. A recent 10-year study at an Eastman

Kodak plant in the United States found that nearly half of those who performed heavy physical labour sought treatment for lower back pain and nearly as many sedentary employees also sought similar treatment. Sedentary white-collar workers suffer back pain because of the long hours that they spend sitting, often in poorly designed chairs; many blue-collar and service workers can blame their back trouble on repeated and improper lifting and carrying.

Why do most backaches occur in the lower back region?
The largest curve in the back is formed by the five vertebrae of the lower spine, which together comprise the lumbar region. These vertebrae, the largest in the spine, support the most weight and are also subject to the greatest strain from such activities as lifting, bending and twisting. These factors make the area much more vulnerable to injury than the relatively inflexible thoracic spine in the middle back and the cervical spine in the neck, which, although more mobile, does not bear as much weight as the lumbar spine.

Can back pain signal other health problems?
Fully 80 to 85 per cent of back pain is muscular in origin, and another 5 to 10 per cent is due to a bulging or ruptured disc. Other back pain may signify an underlying disease or a structural problem. In these cases, back pain can be a symptom of scoliosis, an abnormal sideways curvature of the spine, arthritis or, in rare instances, infections or tumours. Also, backache can signal trouble elsewhere in the body. Kidney and heart disease, as well as prostate, uterine, ovarian, liver and pancreatic problems, may all have back pain as a symptom.

How does poor posture contribute to back problems?
Many experts believe that improper posture places too much stress on the spine. When correctly aligned, the spine curves gently inwards at the neck and lower back, and outwards in the rib area. This modified S shape keeps the head, chest and pelvis centred over one another, balancing the weight of the body. Compromising this posture with rounded shoulders, a slumped sitting position or an excessive arch in the lower back creates weight imbalances that put added strain on the back. Over time, such strain narrows the spaces between the vertebrae. In certain cases, the result is a bulging disc *(see illustration, page 13)*. Fortunately, posture is an area that can be improved dramatically. To evaluate your posture, see pages 22-23. A series of exercises that will help you improve your posture is shown in Chapter Three.

Do sports and other fitness activities help the back?
In general, activity is good for the back. Not only does exercise improve back support, but recent research demonstrates that it directly benefits the discs. A study by an internationally renowned back expert in Sweden showed that exercise aided the flow of nutrients to spinal

discs, possibly delaying their deterioration. Indeed, the only way that discs can receive nutrients is through movement.

Regular exercise is essential for back strength and flexibility; studies have shown that even cardiovascular exercise can improve back problems. However, most popular forms of exercise do little to help strengthen the muscles that support the back. Too often exercises can exert uneven pressure on the back, tightening and straining the muscles as a result. Although there are many cases of professional athletes put out of action by back trouble, most back pain afflicts the novice or weekend athlete, and research has proved that unconditioned exercisers who push far beyond their limits are more likely to injure their backs than are everyday fitness enthusiasts.

If you exercise regularly without back trouble, there is no reason to discontinue doing so. However, you will benefit by adding back-strengthening exercises to your fitness regimen, and making sure that you warm up sufficiently before a workout. If you are subject to back problems, you should avoid certain sports and activities that are likely to aggravate your condition, specifically those that involve lifting, twisting, arching the spine, sudden starts and stops, and falls or collisions. One survey found that 25 per cent of professional golfers suffer from lower back injuries caused by the exertion of twisting. With care, you can modify some of the twisting activities in the sports that encourage back trouble *(see box, page 97)*. Harder to adapt are sports such as rugby and basketball.

Is it true that simply walking upright is the main reason humans have so many back problems?
This is a common misconception that is based on neither evolutionary nor anatomical fact. Indeed, the spine is a marvel of evolution that allowed human beings to walk upright, thereby freeing their hands for more productive use. And walking on four legs is no assurance of a trouble-free back; certain breeds of dogs develop herniated discs. In addition, degenerative arthritis of the spine has been found in birds and reptiles, among other species.

Is sitting all day a major cause of back pain?
Spending too much time sitting in a chair can certainly exacerbate back trouble, especially if your sitting posture is incorrect. A famous Swedish study found that sitting exerted 30 kilograms more pressure on the lower back of a 68-kilogram person than standing did *(see illustration, pages 14-15)*. Slumping does not support the lower back, and hunching your shoulders tenses the neck and upper back muscles. However, sitting properly in well-designed chairs can help.

What other activities create back problems?
Any activity, if performed incorrectly and done repetitively, can weaken the back. Particular offenders are lifting and bending in ways

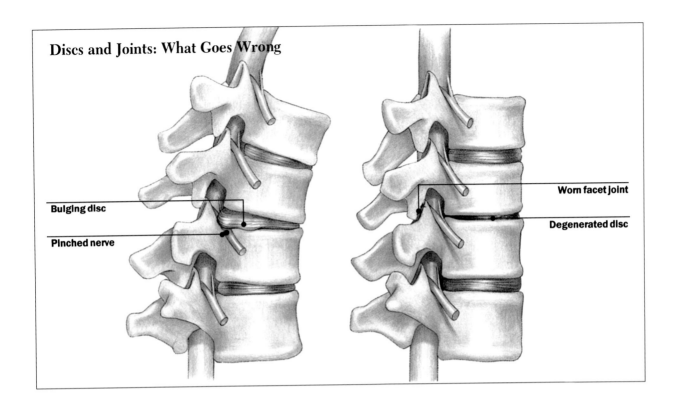

Discs and Joints: What Goes Wrong

Bulging disc

Pinched nerve

Worn facet joint

Degenerated disc

that greatly exaggerate demands on the spine. Comparing lifting with bent knees and lifting with straight knees, the Swedish study noted on page 12 found that the incorrect straight-leg lift places an additional 128 kilograms of stress on the spine. Proper lifting and bending techniques, as well as suggestions for easing strain on the back caused by daily activities, are shown on pages 100-115.

Can backaches be triggered by stress?

Stress can certainly make you vulnerable to back trouble. One recent American study of pain and its relationship to stress found that 46 per cent of respondents reported feelings of stress at least once a week; 35 per cent experienced it less than once a week; and 16 per cent said they never experienced stress. Those with high levels of stress are much more likely to experience all kinds of pain than those with low levels. Sixty-nine per cent of the high-stress group reported backaches in the previous year, as compared with 49 per cent of the group that reported feeling stress once a week or never. One of the physical manifestations of stress is a chronic shortening and tightening of muscles, and many researchers claim that psychological stress can actually trigger muscle spasms. Such back muscle problems can overstretch ligaments and place excess strain on the spine, making it much more prone to injury. Keeping your back muscles flexible with the exercises on pages 56-67 will help alleviate this stress reaction.

Most back pain is muscular in origin, but structural problems with discs and joints are sometimes responsible. Disc problems occur when pressure from surrounding vertebrae causes a disc to bulge *(above, left)* or even rupture. Such deformities can impinge on a nerve, producing intense, radiating pain. As a person ages, discs degenerate, causing them to lose moisture and become thinner. This allows the facet joints to rub against one another *(above, right)*, wearing away their protective coating and causing painful problems such as osteoarthritis. A worn facet joint can also rub directly against nerves and cause pain.

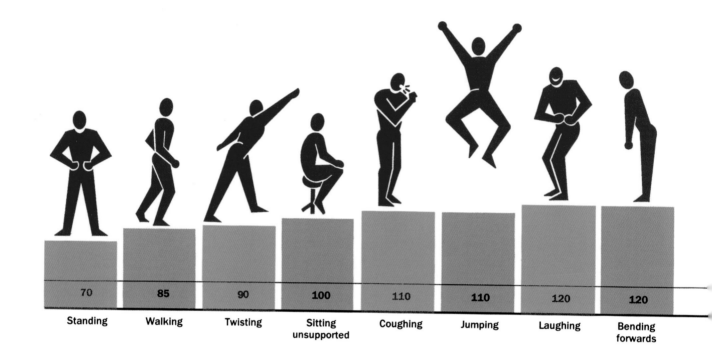

| 70 | 85 | 90 | 100 | 110 | 110 | 120 | 120 |
| Standing | Walking | Twisting | Sitting unsupported | Coughing | Jumping | Laughing | Bending forwards |

How similar are neck pain and lower back pain?

Except for the fact that it is less common and less likely to cause total disability, neck pain is essentially the same as lower back pain. Unfortunately, neck pain, which more often results from a traumatic injury such as whiplash than from general misuse, is not as responsive to exercise treatment as lower back pain is.

Will your back be helped by a specially designed chair or a firmer mattress?

The positions in which you sit and sleep are much more important than what you sit or sleep on. Because everyone's body is different — height, weight, leg length, spinal curvature — sitting and sleeping needs are also individual. Finding the proper chair or mattress for you may take some experimentation. No matter what type of chair you choose, try to find one that you can modify to suit your own back. A well-designed chair adjusts to your height and can accommodate your back needs. If you sleep comfortably on your current mattress, continue to use it; if you do not, first try to improve your sleeping posture, as demonstrated on pages 112-113. Otherwise, you should consider buying a different mattress or using a bedboard.

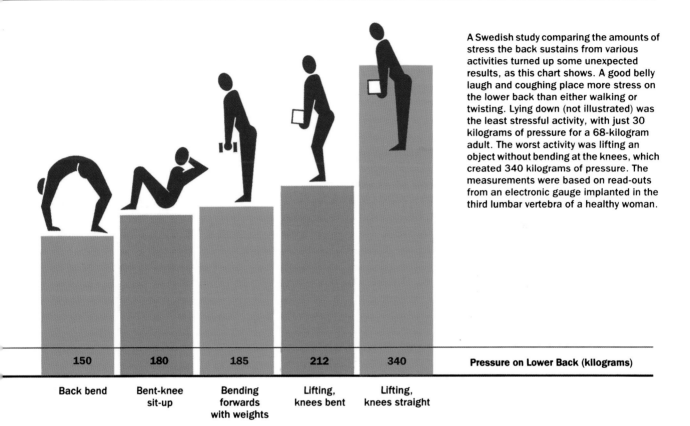

A Swedish study comparing the amounts of stress the back sustains from various activities turned up some unexpected results, as this chart shows. A good belly laugh and coughing place more stress on the lower back than either walking or twisting. Lying down (not illustrated) was the least stressful activity, with just 30 kilograms of pressure for a 68-kilogram adult. The worst activity was lifting an object without bending at the knees, which created 340 kilograms of pressure. The measurements were based on read-outs from an electronic gauge implanted in the third lumbar vertebra of a healthy woman.

150	180	185	212	340	Pressure on Lower Back (kilograms)
Back bend	Bent-knee sit-up	Bending forwards with weights	Lifting, knees bent	Lifting, knees straight	

Does diet have anything to do with your back?

Although back pain strikes the average-weight as well as the over-weight person, there is some evidence that excess weight, particularly in the abdomen, can contribute to back trouble. A potbelly creates the same problem as weak abdominal muscles: both throw off the body's centre of gravity by pulling the lumbar spine forwards into an excessive curve, thus compressing the vertebrae. By maintaining your ideal weight, you will eliminate one contributing factor to back pain. For more information on the connection between your back and your weight, as well as low-fat recipes to help in weight maintenance or reduction, turn to Chapter Five.

What can you do when back pain strikes?

The traditional prescription for backache used to be one to two weeks of bed rest, but recent studies have shown that on average two days is sufficient. This shortened period of bed rest also gives muscles less time to atrophy, which can further complicate back problems. After you have rested and the pain has subsided, stretch your back gently to relieve pressure on the nerves. If severe pain persists after you have spent two days in bed, you should contact your doctor.

Fit Body, Fit Back

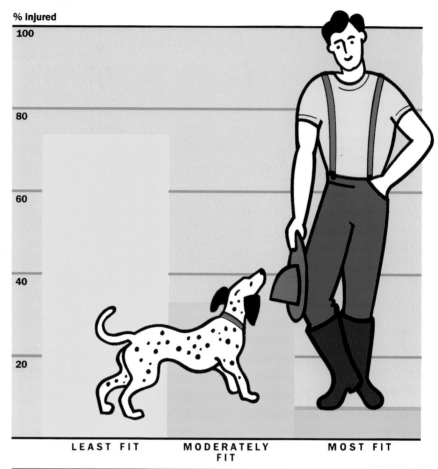

% Injured

A study of 1,652 firemen underscores the importance of fitness for a pain-free back. Based on tests of their cardiovascular endurance, muscular strength and flexibility, the firemen were divided into three groups: most fit, moderately fit and least fit. Researchers traced their back injuries for three years. Back problems were virtually nonexistent among the most fit, while almost 80 per cent of the least fit firemen suffered back injuries.

In conjunction with bed rest, you can take analgesics, such as aspirin or ibuprofen, to reduce both pain and inflammation. In addition, most experts agree that heat can be soothing to muscles in spasm; you should apply it repeatedly for 15 to 20-minute intervals. Although back-care professionals disagree on the value of applying ice to an injured back, the general tendency is to use ice if it seems to help, especially immediately following an injury that affects a local area of the back. Wrapped ice packs should be applied for 10 to 20 minutes every two hours for the first two days.

What is a slipped disc?
In fact, it is a misnomer, because there is no such thing as a "slipped" disc. Discs are firmly anchored between vertebrae and, while they may be subject to considerable degeneration that can create serious problems, they cannot become dislodged. Composed of strong yet flexible fibrous tissue filled with a gelatinous centre, discs play an important role in the spine: by separating the vertebrae, they allow the spine to bend and curve, acting as a shock absorber.

What is often referred to as a slipped disc is actually a disc that has partially collapsed or ruptured as a result of degeneration and strain. When a disc ruptures, or herniates, the outer tissue of the disc tears, allowing the softer material to ooze into the spinal canal. This can lead to severe pain if the disc material presses on a nerve. A bulging, preruptured disc can cause the same sort of pain. However, if the disc never presses on a nerve, you might not even be aware that the condition exists (*see illustration, page 13*). Such a rupture is usually the mechanism behind sciatica, an extremely painful condition that is caused by pressure on the sciatic nerve, which runs along the back of the hip and outer side of the leg.

Fortunately, such disc problems account for only 5 to 10 per cent of all back trouble. And of this percentage, only a small minority require surgery. Up to 90 per cent of those with disc problems respond to the traditional, conservative treatment for back pain: bed rest, analgesics, heat and perhaps physiotherapy. In these cases, rest allows the disc to heal itself by reducing inflammation and reabsorbing the extruded material responsible for the pain.

How long does it take for back pain to subside?

Most back pain subsides within 10 days to three weeks, although the outer limits of this recovery period extend to three months. Only 5 per cent of lower back pain patients have symptoms that persist for more than three months, and even with the more debilitating sciatica, 50 per cent of patients recover within a month.

What is the best way to prevent back trouble?

Studies show that those who are the least physically fit are more likely to have an acute lower back injury than their fitter counterparts. The current consensus among experts is that strengthening and stretching the back with exercises that focus on the back-supporting muscles and, equally important, retraining those muscles to move so as to place the least strain on the back, are the best ways to ensure a healthy back. In addition to its preventive value, regular exercise can diminish chronic pain. Chapter Two of this volume demonstrates back-strengthening exercise routines that match your fitness level.

By keeping your muscles and joints in correct equilibrium, good posture goes hand in hand with strengthening your back. Ways of combining posture and strength to facilitate good back movement day to day are presented in Chapter Four.

It is sometimes possible to avert a bout of back pain if you rest as soon as your back feels fatigued, then gently stretch the back muscles. The Back Attack routine on pages 26-29 is designed to relax muscles by stretching tense muscles and ligaments.

How To Design Your Own Programme

Many people accept back trouble as an inevitable nuisance, but they are doubly mistaken. A bad back is not inevitable, but is often related to your lifestyle or to certain habits that heighten your vulnerability. And if a backache that starts out as just a nuisance is ignored or attended to only intermittently, it can suddenly become very painful.

The questions on the right will help you assess whether you are at particular risk from lower back pain. Once you have answered them, take the simple tests on pages 20-23, which will measure the condition of the muscle groups that offer the most protection against back problems.

Are you a candidate for back trouble?

1 How old are you?

Although back problems can strike adults of virtually any age, the most likely victims are between 30 and 55. During this age span, the spine's discs — which are composed of cartilage and fluid — lose some of their inner moisture and shrink, a phenomenon that partly explains why you may become slightly shorter after you reach middle age. As this degenerative process occurs, either the vertebrae themselves or the facet joints that connect vertebrae to each other may rub together, and such friction is a common cause of backache. After the age of about 55, though, the disc degeneration ceases and the spine assumes a more permanent and rigid configuration that makes it less prone to back disorders, with the exception of osteoarthritis.

2 Have you ever had back pain?

Someone who has had even one episode of back pain is at greater risk than someone who has never experienced such pain: your chances of having a recurrence within two years are about 3 to 2. Unless you have a structural problem in the spine, which can cause recurring back pain, the subsequent episodes can probably be traced to your lifestyle and body mechanics, which include the way you stand, move or lift objects. If your standing and movement patterns strain the muscles in your lower back, you must first become conscious of your bad habits and then try to correct them. You may be able to prevent future attacks by practising good posture, exercising and utilizing other strategies shown in the three following chapters.

3 Are you overweight?

Nearly everyone would like to lose a kilogram or two for appearances' sake. But if you are obese — that is, if you weigh more than 9 kilograms above the ideal weight for a person of your height and build, the excess kilograms may strain your back by creating a gravitational pull on the muscles that support it, especially when the extra weight is carried in the abdomen. Also, overweight people are more likely to be out of shape than their leaner counterparts, and muscle weakness is strongly associated with back problems. A sensible weight-loss programme, combined with muscle-strengthening exercises, will help.

4 How is your posture?

Sway-back posture that exaggerates the normal lumbar, or lower back, curve can be troublesome. Overarching strains the muscles and ligaments in this area, placing undue pressure on the lumbar vertebrae. Contrary to some outdated notions, proper posture does not require a rigidly straight spine, but rather an alignment that follows the spine's natural curves.

5 Are you under a lot of stress?

The precise role that psychological stress plays in causing back problems remains elusive, but many researchers believe that because it creates muscle tension, stress alone can trigger a back attack in some people. If your stress level prevents you from relaxing, muscular tension can occur throughout the body, and particularly in the neck, shoulders and back. Unrelieved tension strains these muscles and decreases their mobility, which may lead to back pain. Research has shown that exercise is an effective stress reliever. A back massage, such as that shown on pages 118-123, can also provide relief.

6 Do you do housework or gardening?

Bending over and pushing a vacuum cleaner, lifting a toddler or straining to reach a high shelf are the occupational hazards of everyday life. Such activities can be just as stressful to the back as heavy labour. A day of raking leaves and gardening can be as hard on the back muscles of an unfit person as several sets of tennis are to a weekend athlete. Shovelling snow, which requires bending, lifting a heavy load and twisting the torso, can also pose serious hazards. Both at home and elsewhere, proper lifting and bending techniques, shown on pages 104-105 and 110-111, can go a long way towards sparing your back.

7 What kinds of exercise do you do?

Muscles need exercise to stay toned and firm; for back care, the muscles of the back, abdomen and thighs should get special attention. The best prescription is for a regular, moderate endurance-exercise programme that gives you an aerobic workout three times a week for 20 minutes or more, combined with the special back-care exercises in Chapter Two.

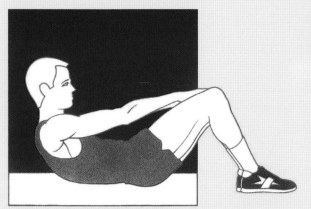

Abdominals/1: Lie with your knees bent. Tilt your pelvis back to flatten your lower back. With your arms outstretched, lift your shoulders and upper back. If you cannot hold this position for at least 30 seconds, your abdominal strength is poor.

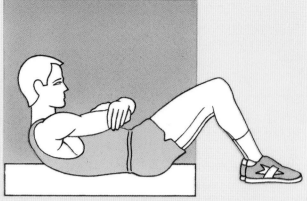

Abdominals/2: Start in the same position as for the previous exercise, but this time cross your arms over your chest. Lift your upper back off the floor and hold. If you can maintain this position for at least 30 seconds, your abdominal strength is fair.

How Strong Is Your Back?

As with any fitness programme, the best approach to conditioning your back is progressive: if your back-supporting muscles are weak, they must be strengthened gradually. While the basic back exercises in this volume are gentle enough for almost anyone without acute back pain, the advanced routines are designed for those who are quite fit. Do not attempt the more rigorous exercises before you have built up adequate muscular strength. Excessive zeal at any point in an exercise programme can put you out of action.

The exercises on these two pages evaluate the strength of the muscles that are most vital for supporting your back — your abdominals, back extensors and quadriceps. Basing your calculations on the amount of time you can sustain each exercise, you will be able to rate your back strength as poor, fair, good or excellent. The four sit-up variations given above test your abdominals progressively; if you can do the first, advance to the second, third or fourth. Evaluate your quadriceps strength with the wall slide on the right, and test your back extensors with the back lift on the far right.

The results of these strength tests will steer you to the most suitable exercises in Chapter Two. If you are in the poor category, start with the basic routines on pages 40-45. If your rating is fair, turn to the moderate strengtheners on pages 46-51. And if your muscle strength rates either good or excellent, you can try the advanced routine on pages 52-55.

If you fall into more than one category — say you are good on the abdominals test but poor on the back-extensor test — choose the easier routine instead of combining basic and intermediate exercises. It is important to let your weaker muscles catch up, thereby developing a full support system for your back.

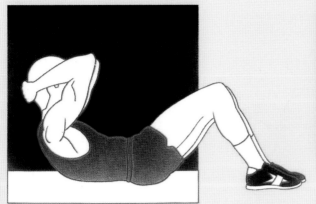

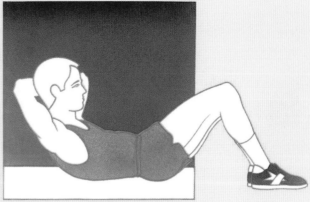

Abdominals/3: From the same starting position, clasp your hands behind your neck, keeping your arms close by your head as you raise your upper back. (Do not assist the movement by pulling your head.) Holding for at least 30 seconds indicates that your abdominal strength is good.

Abdominals/4: Clasp your hands behind your neck, this time keeping your elbows out to the sides as you lift your upper back. (Do not assist the movement by pulling your head.) If you can hold this position for at least 30 seconds, the strength of your abdominal muscles is excellent.

Quadriceps: With your back against a wall and your feet about half a metre in front of you, slide down so your thighs and calves form a 45 to 90-degree angle. Holding for 30 seconds is fair. Less than 30 seconds is poor; longer is good.

Back extensors: Lie face down with your arms at your sides. Raise your head and chest; hold. If you can sustain this position for one minute, your strength is fair; less than this amount of time is considered poor, and longer is good.

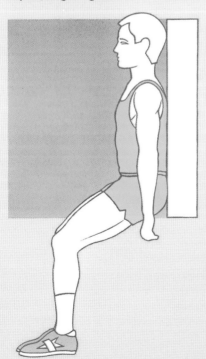

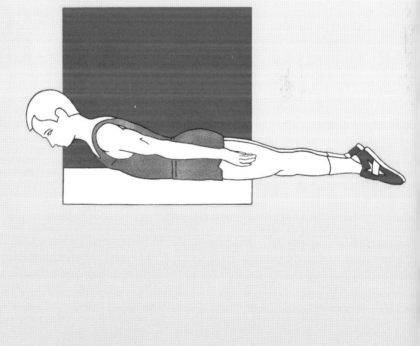

Is Your Posture a Problem?

Posture plays an important role in back care. Aligning your spine correctly allows your abdominal and back muscles to support the back with optimal effectiveness. Incorrect alignment, however, strains certain muscles while leaving others underused. Thus, postural improvements should always accompany back-strengthening exercises for the exercises to be effective.

Evaluating your posture as shown on the right is the first step towards improving it. Stand sideways in front of a mirror in your natural posture, either nude, or wearing form-fitting exercise clothes. Compare your own alignment to the standing image. Then sit sideways in front of the mirror and make the same comparison. You will have to turn your head, but doing this will not disrupt your posture from the neck down.

Another way of evaluating how you stand is to check the soles of your shoes for the patterns of wear, as indicated below.

If your posture departs from the ideals shown on the right, perform the exercises on pages 72-93, which are designed to encourage changes in long-standing postural habits.

Look at the sole of an exercise or walking shoe you have worn for at least a few weeks. Any wear patterns similar to those shown on the right indicate faulty posture. Excess wear on the inside of your shoe is due to pronation, an inward rotation of the foot. On the outside of the soles, wear is from supination, an outward rotation. While the proper shoes may alleviate some rotation problems, postural improvements can provide more lasting benefits.

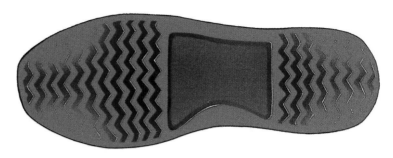

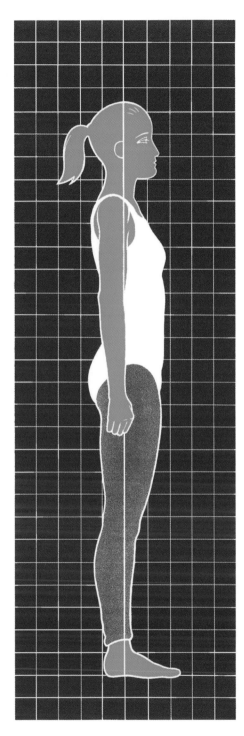

When standing in front of a mirror *(left)*, imagine that a plumb line has been dropped through the centre of your head through the front of your earlobe, the front of your shoulder, the centre of your hip, behind your kneecap and in front of your anklebone. There should be gentle inward curves at your neck and lower back, and a gentle outward curve at your upper back.

When you are sitting *(below)*, the plumb line should pass through the same points and out of the centre of your hip. There should not be an excessive curve in your lower back.

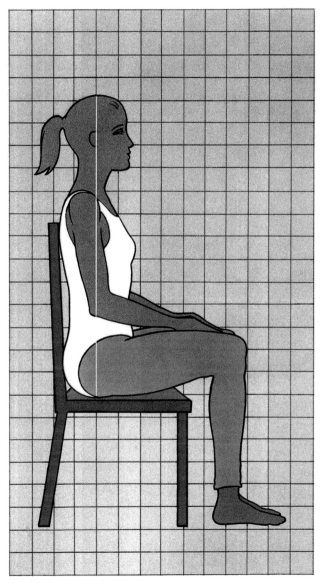

Help for a Bad Back

The vast majority of back-pain victims are relieved to learn that the trouble is muscular and responds to simple, readily available therapies: bed rest, aspirin and, finally, an exercise programme of stretching and strengthening. For a small minority of sufferers, though, other forms of treatment are essential. The chart below lists some of the choices, from braces and supports, a basic treatment, to surgery, the most risky.

You should consult a doctor if you have a backache that does not improve after two days of bed rest, coupled with aspirin or ibuprofen taken every four hours. Your doctor will examine you to verify that you have no structural problem or disease. If it is necessary for you to see a medical specialist, your doctor may refer you to an orthopaedic specialist who treats problems of the muscles

Back Treatment Guide

ACUPUNCTURE	This traditional Chinese treatment, which involves inserting thin needles in the body at certain points, offers relief to some sufferers: in one survey, 54 per cent of those undergoing acupuncture reported less pain. Western doctors now understand how acupuncture works: the needles encourage the release of chemicals which are part of the body's natural defence system. These act as painkillers and initiate the process of self-healing within the body.
BRACES AND SUPPORTS	Corsets, braces and back supports can be helpful during the acute stages of back pain, or they may serve as a preventive measure if you are prone to back problems and know you are in for a physically demanding day. These items support your back and maintain your posture. Ultimately, however, muscles should be doing this job, and using artificial support for long periods weakens the muscles, so the treatment becomes self-defeating.
DRUGS	If the pain is severe, your doctor may prescribe a strong painkiller such as codeine, plus an aspirin or other anti-inflammatory drug. The newer types of anti-inflammatory drugs have often proved no more effective than aspirin or a combination of aspirin and codeine, while producing more side effects. Some doctors also prescribe muscle relaxants, such as Valium. Since these compounds and some painkillers have a sedative effect, keep your activity to a minimum while you are taking them. At most, the drugs will lessen the pain during the acute phase of an attack. Some drugs are addictive and doctors are reluctant to prescribe them for long periods.
ELECTRICAL STIMULATION	Also called TENS for Transcutaneous Electrical Nerve Stimulation, this treatment sends mild electrical current to contracted muscle areas, or "trigger points", that send pain radiating to other sites. A tiny battery-powered TENS device can be worn under your clothing, and you can activate it when pain strikes. Although its effects are not comprehended fully, the temporary relief that TENS provides may be due to the ability of the electrical current to interfere with the body's pain perception mechanisms. (Manual stimulation of trigger points is demonstrated on pages 116-117.)
GRAVITY BOOTS AND INVERSION DEVICES	Hanging upside down in gravity boots or another kind of inversion system is a kind of traction, and some back-pain sufferers find it relaxing. Some proponents suggest that by widening the space between the vertebrae, inversion relieves pressure on the spinal discs. However, because the upside-down position elevates blood pressure and may increase pressure in the eyes, it should be avoided by anyone with hypertension or glaucoma, and should only ever be done under careful supervision.

and bones; a physiotherapist, who practises rehabilitative medicine; or a neurologist, who is an expert in nerve disorders.

For a muscular problem that does not respond to rest and aspirin or another analgesic, you might want to consult a chiropractor, a non-medical specialist who diagnoses pain and muscular disorders as manifestations of spinal misalignments, and treats conditions with manipulation. Other non-medical specialists who treat back problems include both massage therapists and acupuncturists.

If your back pain persists after you have tried a variety of treatments, you may want to explore services offered by a pain clinic. These centres help people to cope with persistent, intractable pain by using such approaches and techniques as biofeedback, visualization, psychotherapy, meditation and hypnosis.

INJECTIONS	Doctors sometimes inject anti-inflammatory drugs, most commonly cortisone, or local anaesthetics into the sore muscles of back-pain victims who have not responded to more conservative treatments. Cortisone injections can be beneficial for severe pain, and some doctors believe that anaesthetics can break the pain cycle and relieve spasm when injected into the affected muscle. Some patients have gained relief when their ruptured discs are injected with an enzyme derived from papaya. Called chymopapain, the enzyme may be able to dissolve the protruding part of the disc.
MANUAL THERAPIES	Back-pain victims who responded to a recent survey reported that both massage and chiropractic manipulation produced significant, if temporary, relief. Swedish massage, which involves soothing, gliding motions, helped 66 per cent of those who tried it. Shiatsu, Japanese pressure-point therapy which works deeper in the muscles, helped 79 per cent, including some who found little relief elsewhere. (A home massage routine is shown on pages 118-123.) Chiropractic manipulation of the spine aided 56 per cent. In another study of back-pain sufferers divided into two groups, 50 per cent of the group who underwent chiropractic manipulation were pain-free a week after treatment, compared with 27 per cent of those treated with bed rest and painkillers. However, doctors warn that you should not receive treatment from a chiropractor if you have a ruptured or herniated disc; sciatica, a nerve problem that affects the legs, hips and buttocks; or any disease of the spine.
SURGERY	Today surgery is generally advised for fewer than 5 per cent of sufferers, and then only as a last resort. Even ruptured discs frequently heal without surgery, according to a number of studies. Typically, surgery is undertaken only if a ruptured disc or bone spur impinges far enough on a nerve to cause sciatic leg pain with accompanying numbness and muscular weakness.
TRACTION	When you are placed in traction a mechanical apparatus that may include harnesses, straps, pulleys and weights in effect pulls the upper and lower parts of your body in opposite directions. Traction stretches the back muscles and ligaments, and some proponents believe that it opens up space for the discs. Although most people are hospitalized to undergo traction, a number of devices are designed for home use. As a rule, this therapy provides short-term relief, and once you stop using traction, your vertebrae will gradually return to their former positions.

Dealing with Back Attacks

Episodes of back spasm are usually immobilizing as well as painful; once they strike, there is not much that you can do but lie down. Fortunately, while some attacks come on suddenly, most attacks are preceded by telltale twinges and excessive back fatigue. In fact, except for traumatic injury, nearly all back spasms mark the culmination of problems that have been growing worse for some time. Learning to respond to your back's signals can help to prevent fully fledged spasms before they develop.

The sequence that follows is designed to prevent or reduce pain by relaxing your back-supporting muscles and lengthening your spine, thus relieving compression of the vertebrae. When you do experience back pain, first lie down to eliminate the pressure on the spine. After a period of rest, gentle stretching will help to relax back muscles and take pressure off the nerves.

These exercises should be done slowly and gently. They are designed to help your back feel better; do not perform any movement that causes pain. If your back pain is so severe that you cannot perform any of these exercises, consult your doctor.

The two exercises demonstrated on page 29 can be performed when back pain strikes and you have nowhere to lie down to recuperate. By reducing the curve in your lower back, they relieve pressure from too much standing or walking.

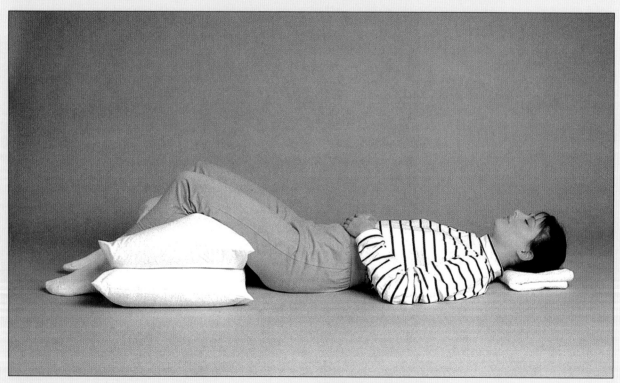

Whenever your back bothers you, this position is ideal for resting and relieving pressure on your spine. Place a small pillow or rolled-up towel under your head to prevent it from tipping back. Raise your knees by putting one or two large pillows underneath to keep your back flat. Close your eyes and relax for at least 20 minutes before continuing the sequence.

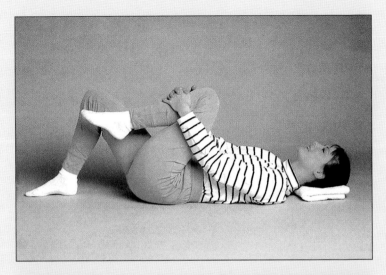

Leave the small pillow or towel under your head. Remove the large pillows but keep your knees bent. Grasp your left knee with both hands and pull it gently towards your chest. Lower and repeat with your other leg.

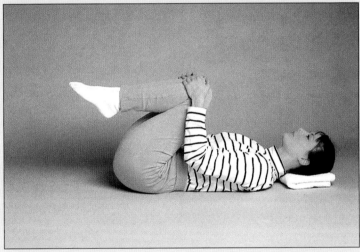

Remain lying down with both knees bent and your feet flat on the floor. Keeping your back flat, grasp your knees and gently pull them towards your chest. Lower your knees.

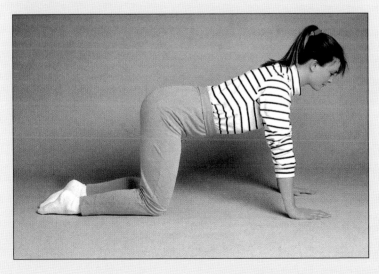

Carefully roll over on to your stomach and raise yourself on to your hands and knees, with your arms shoulder-width apart and your knees hip-width apart. Then gently arch your back.

27

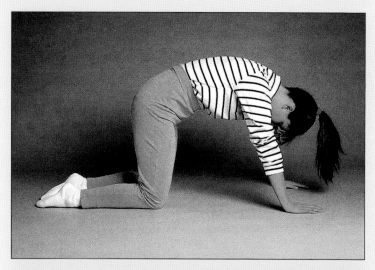

Stay on your hands and knees and drop your head between your arms. Round your back, allowing it to curve upwards.

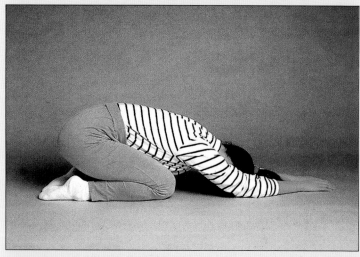

With your legs about 5 centimetres apart, lower your buttocks to your heels, folding your chest on to your thighs and dropping your forehead to the floor. Keep your arms extended in front of your head.

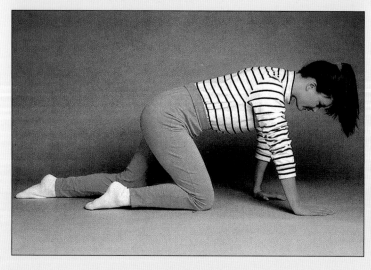

Keep your head down and your neck and back straight and raise yourself on to your hands and knees. Using alternate arms and legs, crawl a metre or two forwards, then retrace your movement backwards.

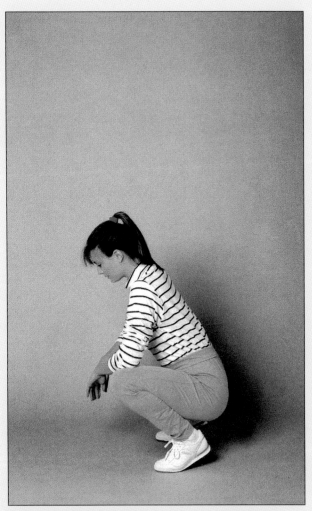

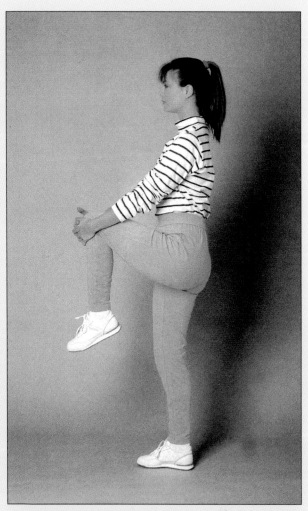

From an upright position, lower yourself into a squat, if necessary resting your heels on a book. Keep your back and neck aligned and rest your elbows on your knees. Hold for approximately 30 seconds.

From a standing position, bend your left leg and raise it to hip height or higher. Clasp your hands round your knee and pull the leg towards your chest slightly. Hold for several seconds; lower and repeat with the other leg.

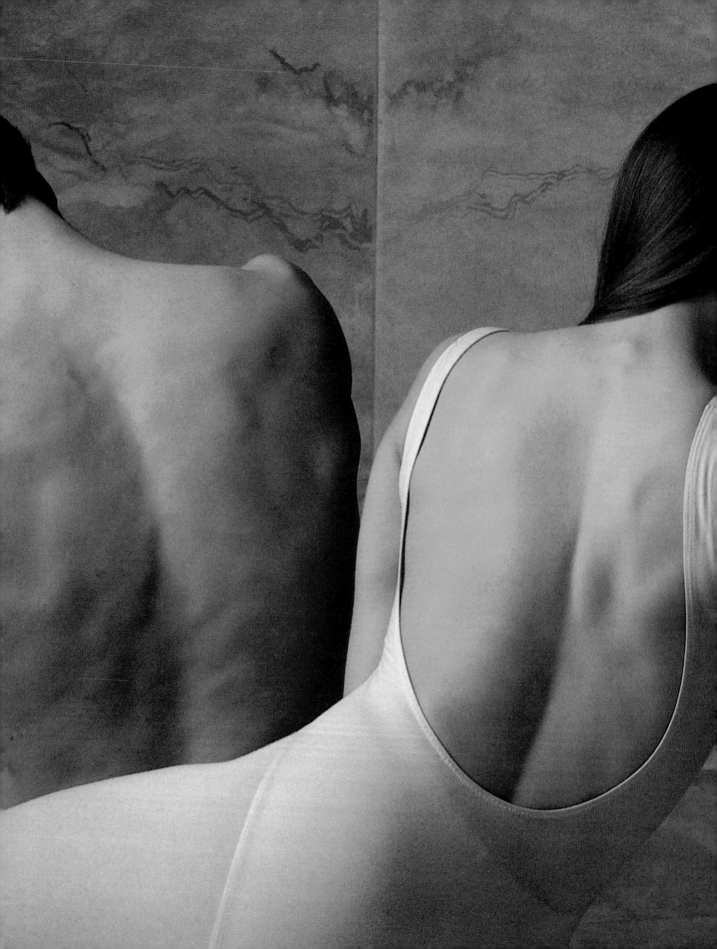

CHAPTER TWO

Building a Better Back

*A progressive strengthening
and stretching routine
for insurance against backache*

T he principle that strong, flexible muscles are the best defence against most types of injury proves especially valid where the back is concerned. An exercise programme aimed at strengthening all the muscles that support the back is one effective step you can take to prevent lower back problems.

Research has confirmed that the majority of back-pain sufferers can blame their discomfort on muscular weaknesses. In one study, only 17 per cent of a group of back-pain patients showed signs of structural problems or pathology. But when the entire group of 3,000 people were given six standard tests to measure the strength and flexibility of the muscles that support the back, 83 per cent of them failed one or more tests. In a separate study of 174 patients who had made significant improvements in the same tests, 88 per cent reported a decrease in back pain accompanying the muscular changes.

Several recent studies have shown that the proper type of exercises, when performed regularly, can contribute to restoring strength and flexibility in a back that has been injured or weakened by strain, sprain or spasm. One such study in the United States involved 12,000 men and women enrolled in a YMCA programme to combat lower back pain. Working out both at home and at their local YMCA, participants engaged daily in strengthening, relaxation and flexibility exercises for six weeks. Four out of five — including those who had suffered back pain for up to 15 years — reported that their pain had vanished or was alleviated by the end of the programme. Whether a participant had previously tried another form of treatment had no significant impact on any improvement that occurred. Of the nearly 600 participants who had undergone back surgery but enrolled because of continuing pain, those who exercised daily for more than half an hour showed more dramatic improvement than those who worked out less often.

Exercises targeted at strengthening the back focus on three groups of muscles. The abdominals, latissimus dorsi and obliques support the torso itself. The erector spinae muscles, called the back extensors, extend the length of the spine and connect to the vertebrae, providing direct support and stability for the spine. The quadriceps, the large four-part muscles along the fronts of the thighs, stabilize the pelvis.

Of these muscle groups, the abdominals are the most important for back support, functioning much like powerful rubber bands to connect your upper and lower body and transfer force between them. When well conditioned, these muscles, which run diagonally, horizontally and vertically, create the equivalent of a muscular girdle that protects the internal organs and keeps the lower back from over-arching into a sway-back position. Aerobic workouts, weight training and other forms of exercise often fail to condition the abdominals. One study of Canadian athletes who competed in the 1976 Olympics found that they had relatively weak abdominal muscles. Some of them were unable to perform more than one bent-knee sit-up.

Weak abdominal muscles put the back in double jeopardy. Not only do lax abdominals fail to provide adequate support but, because they are less able to resist the pull of the body's weight on the spine, they may actually create strain in your back. Although they are not designed for the task of keeping your spine upright, the spinal muscles are forced to assume most of the burden. Performing abdominal-strengthening exercises will help alleviate this overload on the spine.

Strong back extensors can absorb much of the stress of everyday movements such as leaning forwards. However, these key muscles tend to be misused in people who suffer chronic back trouble. The lack of torso support from weak abdominals is often compensated for by the extensors. Similarly, the back extensors are commonly used for lifting — a function more appropriately relegated to the quadriceps. Such inappropriate demands stress the extensors, making them prone to sprain, which can result in painful backaches.

The quadriceps, among the largest and most powerful muscles in the body, supply much of the momentum for running, jumping and all

Muscles that Maintain Your Back

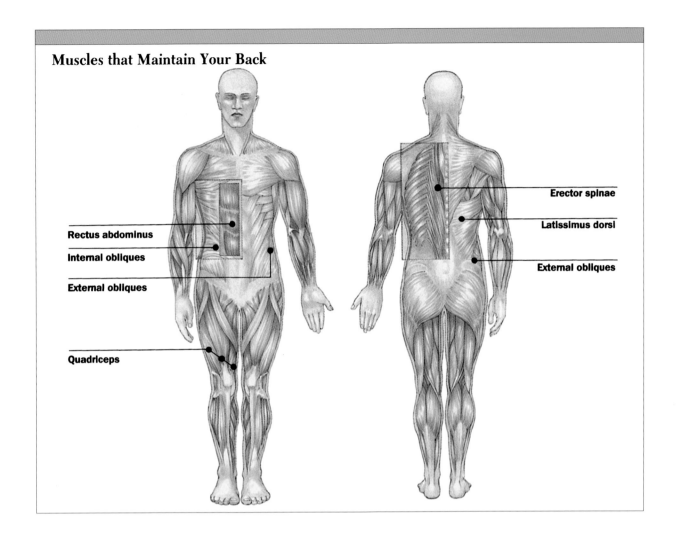

Rectus abdominus

Internal obliques

External obliques

Quadriceps

Erector spinae

Latissimus dorsi

External obliques

other forms of forward movement. When appropriately used, they have the capacity to relieve the back of much of the burden of lifting heavy objects. Lifting and bending should utilize the quadriceps, rather than the muscles of the back. Strengthening your quadriceps will allow you to use them more comfortably for lifting.

Doctors advise that you should not begin an exercise programme if you are suffering intense or disabling back pain. Wait until the injured tissues have had a chance to heal; exercise may aggravate the problem rather than relieve it. The following workout includes both strengthening and flexibility exercises. The strengthening sequence is divided into basic, moderate and advanced exercises. If you have not exercised regularly for some time, start with the minimal number of repetitions. Do not advance to the next level until you can comfortably perform the maximum number. Be aware of how your back adapts itself to the exercises and stop if you feel any pain. Always work slowly and smoothly, avoiding sudden jerking movements. For the best results, perform the range-of-motion and stretching exercises daily, and the strengthening exercises at least three times a week.

Range of Motion Routine/1

Building strength in the back requires a comprehensive fitness programme aimed at increasing both muscle strength and muscle flexibility, as well as maximizing range of motion within the joints. The exercises in this chapter target all three of these areas.

The exercises are intended to be performed as a whole routine. The warm-up consists of the range-of-motion sequences on these two pages and the following four. These exercises enhance flexibility in the hip joints, which connect the pelvis to the legs, as well as in the vertebrae themselves. Strengthening and stretching sequences make up the remainder of the chapter.

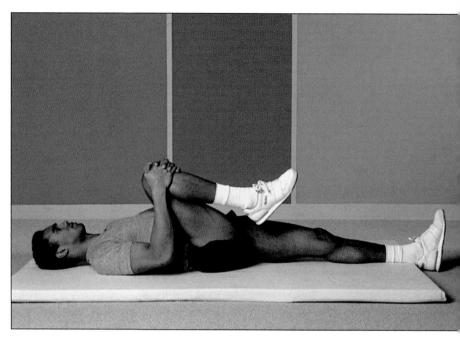

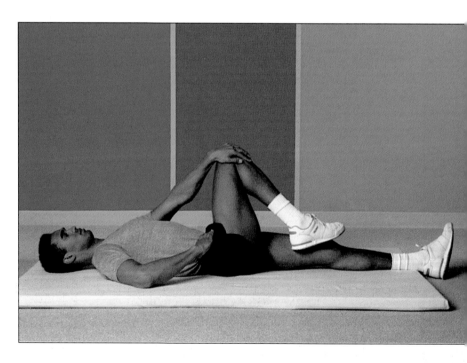

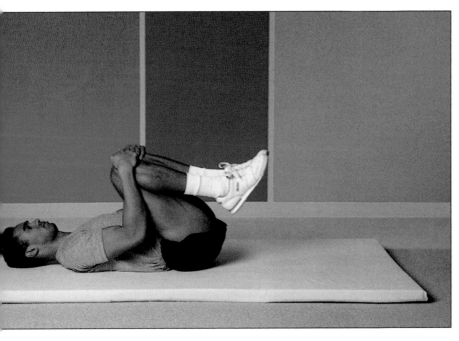

To increase hip joint range of motion, lie on your back with your legs extended. Bend your right knee and grasp it with your hands, bringing it towards your chest *(far left)*. Hold for 10 seconds, then lower. Repeat three to five times with the right knee. Switch knees and repeat. Then bring up both knees and grasp them for 10 seconds *(left)*; lower. Repeat three to five times.

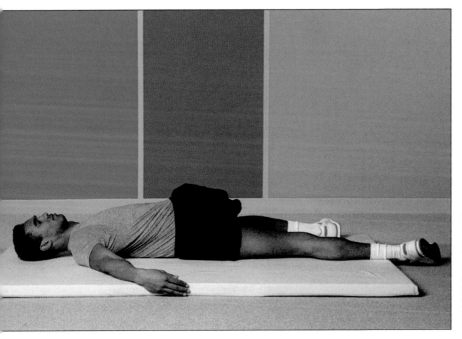

Lying down with your legs extended, bend your right knee so that your right foot touches your left knee. Place your right hand at your right hip to make sure it is flat and grasp your right knee with your other hand *(far left)*. Next, keeping your shoulders flat, rotate your right hip as you pull your knee across your body with your left hand *(left)*. Hold for 10 seconds, return and repeat three to five times. Switch legs and repeat.

Range of Motion
Routine/2

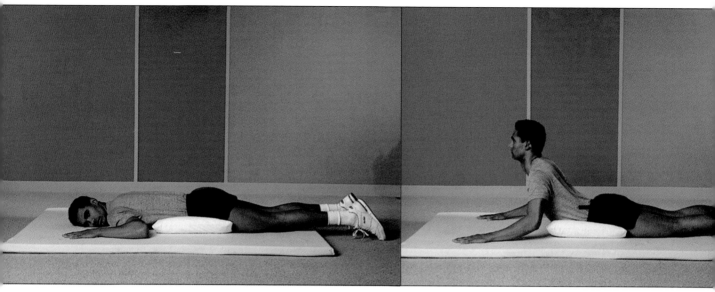

To improve the range of motion in your lower back, lie on your abdomen with a pillow beneath you and your elbows bent so that your hands are about 15 centimetres in front of your shoulders *(above)*. Pushing up with your arms, raise your upper body so that it curves gently to form a "C" *(above, right)*. Keep your elbows slightly bent. Lower. Perform 10 repetitions.

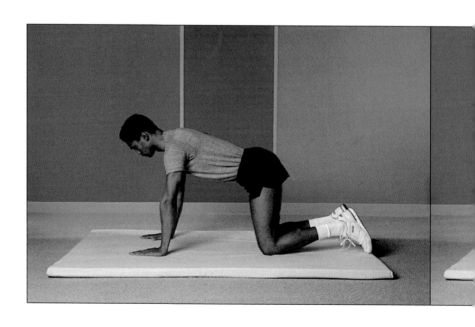

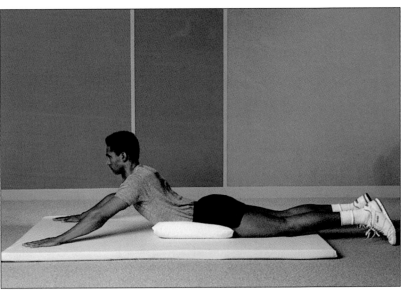

If the exercise opposite causes pain, try this variation. Place your hands 30 centimetres in front of your shoulders and push up, straightening your arms.

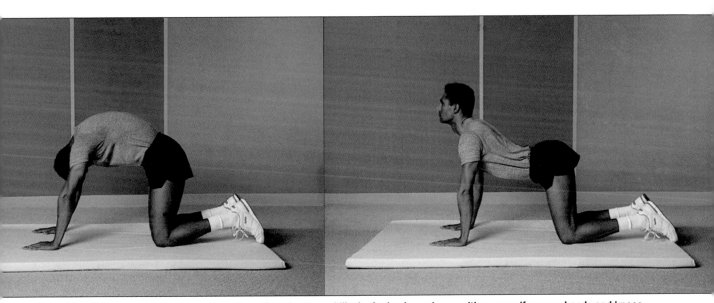

To enhance mobility in the lumbar spine, position yourself on your hands and knees with your back flat *(above, left)*. Shift your weight slightly backwards, tucking your head and rounding your back upwards *(above, centre)*. Then shift your weight forwards, arching your back and lifting your head *(above)*. Hold each position for 10 seconds and repeat the sequence five times.

Range of Motion Routine/3

For greater mobility in the thoracic spine, rest on your knees and forearms, with your entire spine straight, including the neck *(right)*. Shift your weight forwards, arching your back slightly *(centre)*. Then shift your weight backwards, rounding your back and dropping your head *(bottom)*. Hold each position for 10 seconds; repeat five times.

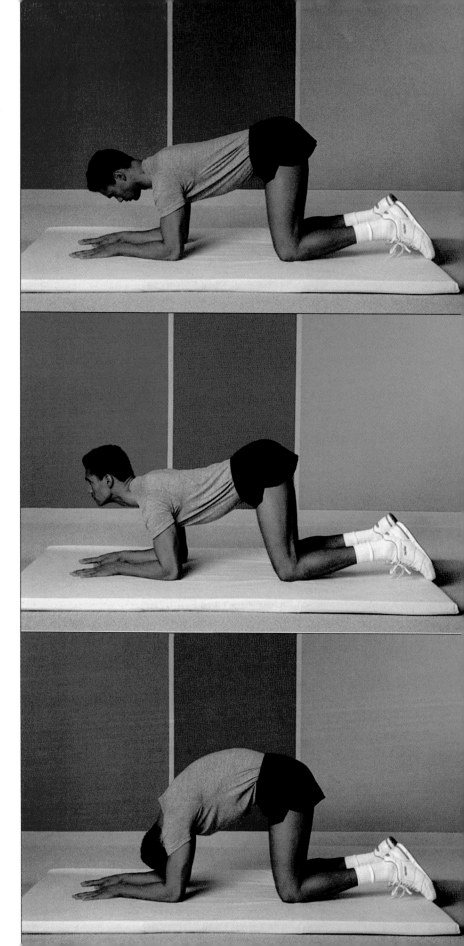

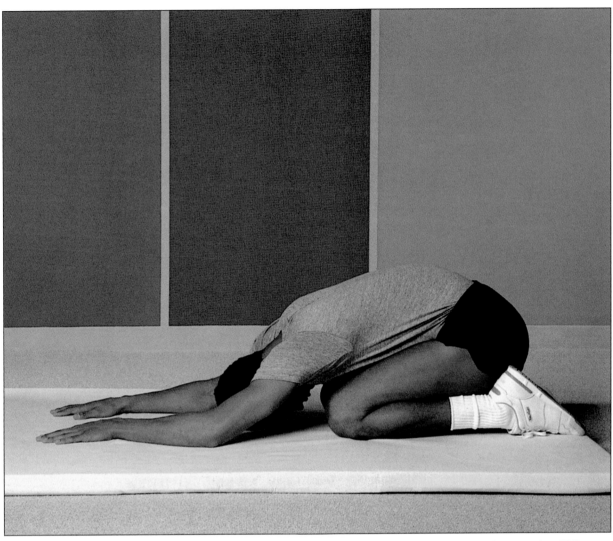

Kneel with your legs together. Shift your weight backwards trying to rest your buttocks on your heels. Then tuck your head and drop your chest to your thighs *(above)*. Keep your arms extended in front of you. Hold for up to 30 seconds.

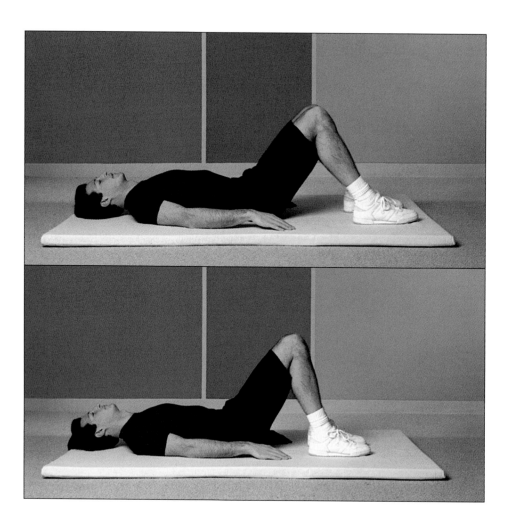

Strengtheners and Stretches

Maximizing both the strength and flexibility of the back-supporting musculature is the basis of back fitness. The major muscles supporting the back are the back extensors and latissimus dorsi in the back, the abdominal muscles, and the quadriceps at the front of the thigh (see box, page 33).

The exercises in the remainder of this chapter focus on these muscle groups. The strengthening exercises are divided into three groups: basic, intermediate and advanced. Unless you were in the highest performance categories on the strong-back test on pages 20-21, you should probably start with the basic routine. Even if you are generally quite fit, your back-supporting musculature will be weak unless you have targeted it in a training programme.

If you experience pain while performing these exercises, reduce the repetitions or drop back a level. When more than one set is indicated, pause for 15 to 30 seconds between sets. Particularly at the advanced level, these exercises are quite rigorous. The routines will strengthen your back and tone your midsection, making you look slimmer.

Complete your back workout with the stretching routine demonstrated on pages 56-61 and the three neck stretches on pages 62-65.

BASIC STRENGTHENERS: To tighten your upper abdominals, lie on your back with your knees bent and your arms at your sides *(top)*. Rotate your pelvis back, flattening your lower back against the floor to tilt your abdomen upwards *(above)*. Focus on the muscles involved, being careful not to tighten your buttocks or lift your ribs. Do two sets of 10, holding for five seconds each.

For lower abdominal strength, lie flat on your back with your arms at your sides *(opposite, above)*. Raise your head and lift your arms, rounding your upper back *(opposite)*. You should feel your lower abdominals contract. Hold for five seconds; repeat 10 times.

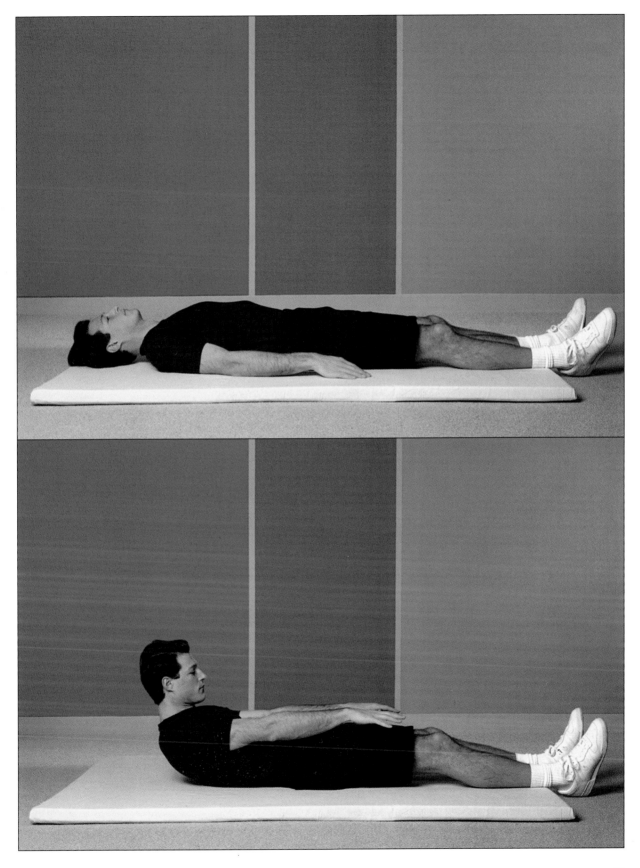

Basic
Strengtheners/2

To strengthen the oblique abdominals, which run diagonally, bend your knees while lying on your back. Lift your legs and cross your feet. Cross your hands behind your head *(right)*. Twist your left elbow towards your right knee, raising your upper back *(centre)*; lower yourself back down. Twist up again to raise your right elbow towards your left knee *(bottom)*. Work up to three sets of 10.

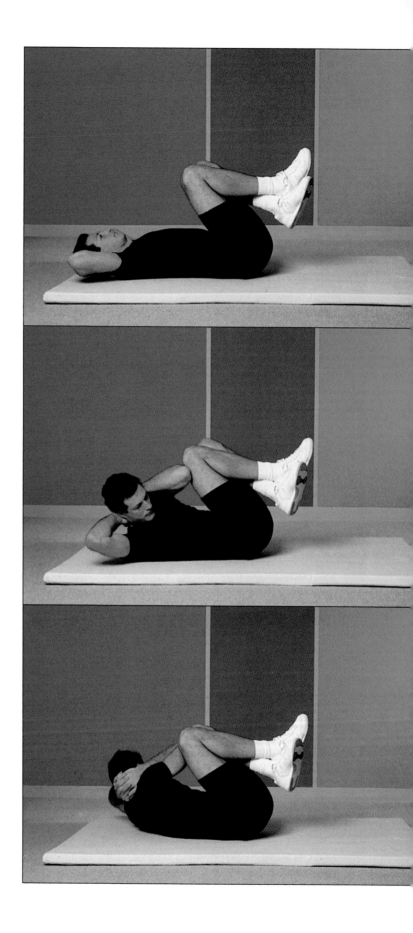

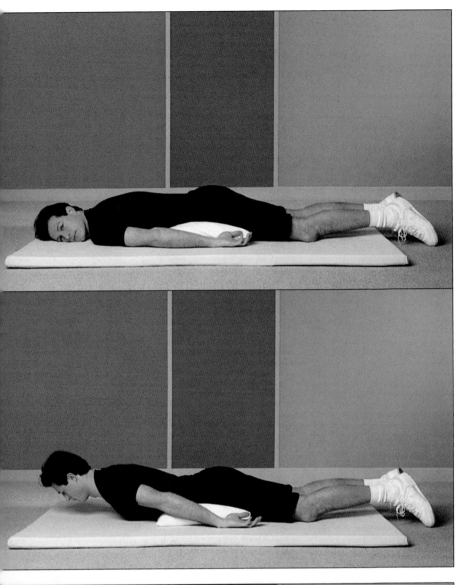

To strengthen your back muscles,
lie prone with a pillow beneath your
abdomen and your arms at your sides
(above). Squeeze your shoulders together
to bring your upper body up slightly *(left)*.
Keep your neck in line with your spine;
lower yourself back down. Perform 10
full repetitions.

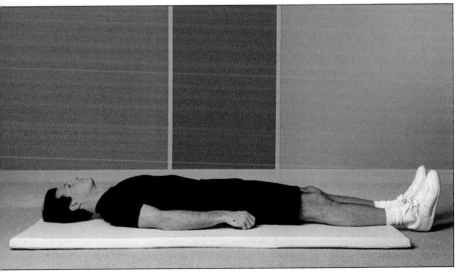

To build up the thigh muscles needed for
proper lifting, lie on your back with your
arms at your sides. Tighten the quadriceps,
or thigh muscles, of your left leg as much
as possible *(left)*. Perform 10 repetitions
holding for 10 seconds each. Switch legs
and repeat.

Basic
Strengtheners/3

This exercise uses the test for quadriceps strength on page 20 to build up these muscles. Stand with your back, shoulders and buttocks flat against a wall *(right)*. Move your heels about 30 centimetres from the wall. Slide down the wall, keeping your back flat, until your knees and thighs are at about a 45-degree angle *(centre)*. Stop at this point if your knees hurt; otherwise continue sliding down until your legs form a 90-degree angle *(far right)*. Hold your position for 15 seconds; rise and repeat twice. To increase the difficulty, build up to sets of 60 seconds in 10-second increments.

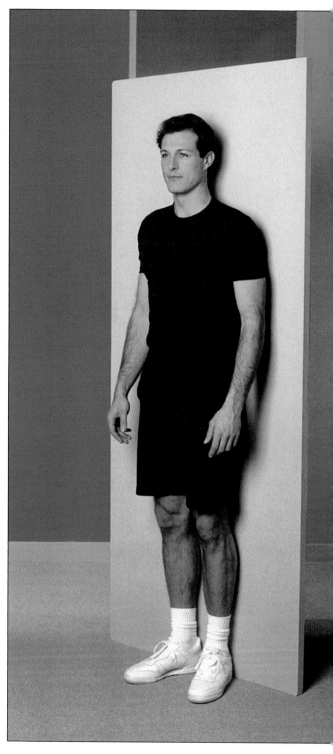

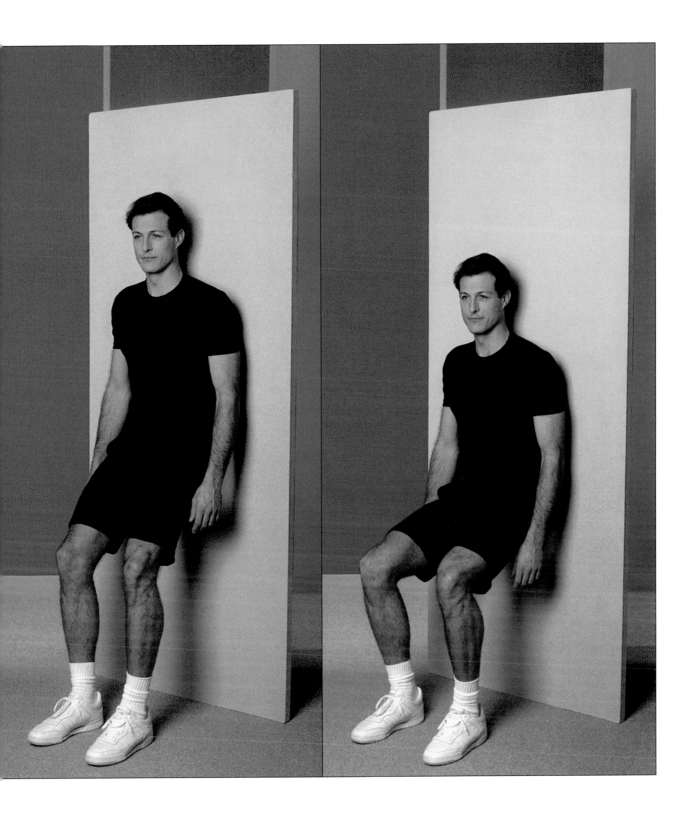

Intermediate Strengtheners/1

To further increase abdominal strength, lie on your back with your knees bent and your feet flat on the floor *(right)*. Bend your elbows, place your hands at your temples and, keeping your elbows close together, lift your upper back so that your shoulder blades come off the mat *(far right)*. Do three sets of 10, eventually working up to sets of 20 repetitions.

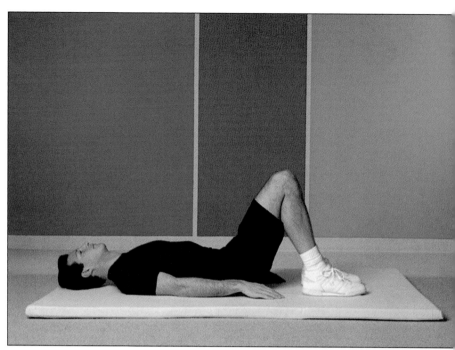

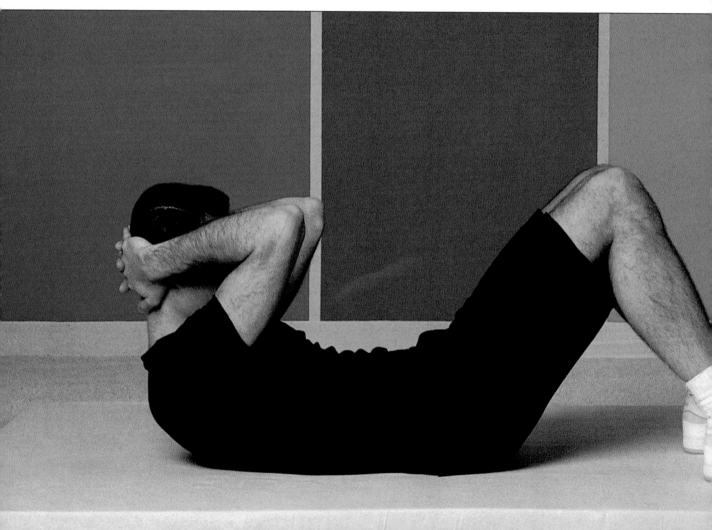

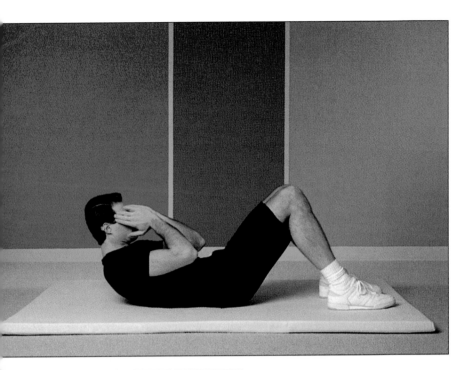

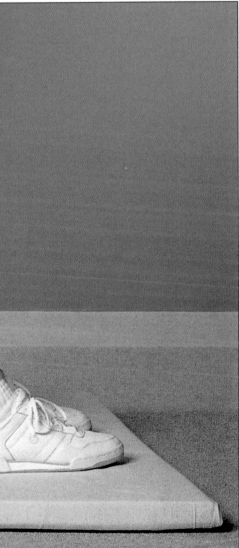

If you have any neck pain, do this variation on the above exercise: clasp your hands behind your neck for support, keeping your elbows close by your head. Raise your shoulders off the mat, taking care not to pull on your neck.

Intermediate Strengtheners/2

Improve lower abdominal strength by lying on your back with your left knee bent and left foot on the floor, your right knee raised towards your chest *(right)*. Straighten your right knee, pointing the sole of your foot towards the ceiling *(centre)*. Slowly lower your right leg, stopping just before your back begins to arch *(bottom)*. Keep your hips down. Hold for 10 seconds; return to the starting position. It is important to keep your back flat. Perform 10 repetitions for each leg.

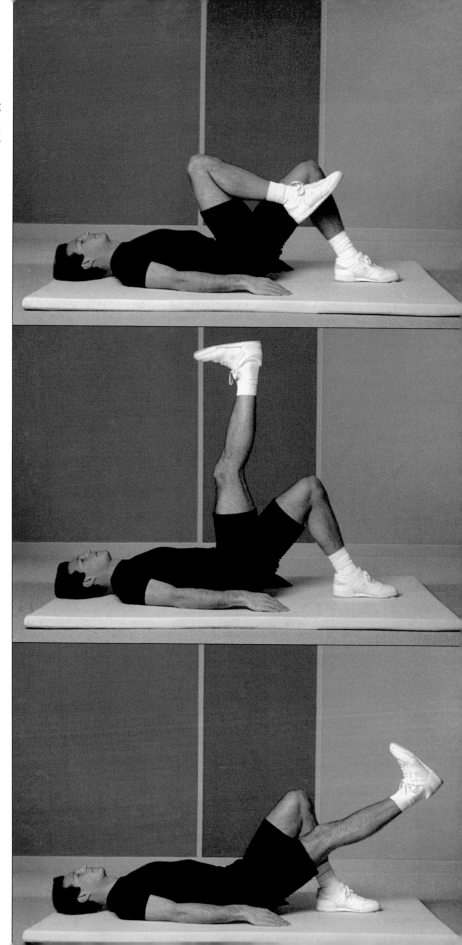

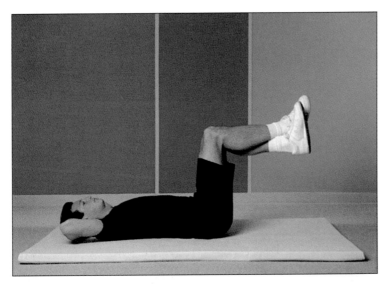

To strengthen the oblique abdominals, lie flat on your back with your legs raised and knees bent to form a 90-degree angle. Cross your ankles and cross your hands under your head *(left)*. Lift your upper back and twist to your right, reaching your left elbow to your right knee *(below)*. Lower and twist to your left. Perform three sets of 10 repetitions.

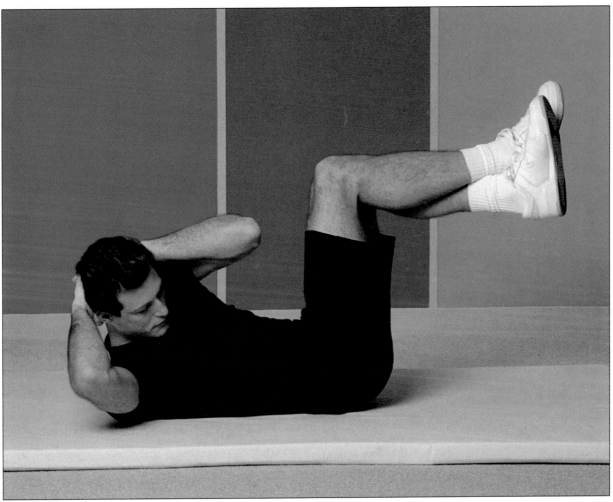

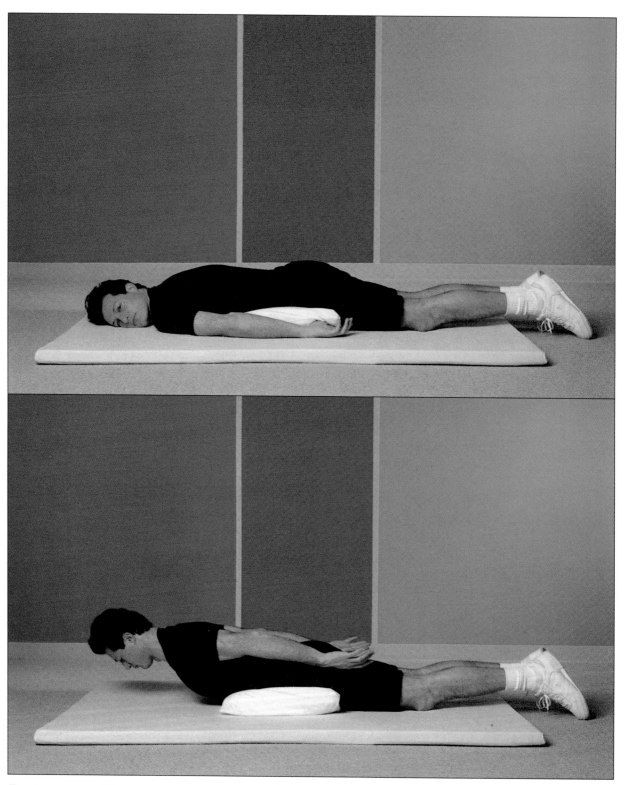

Intermediate
Strengtheners/3

Increase the strength of your back muscles by lying prone with your arms at your sides and a pillow beneath you *(top)*. Lift your upper back, raising your arms and your entire upper torso *(above)*. Keep your head in line with your spine. Do two sets of 10 repetitions.

50

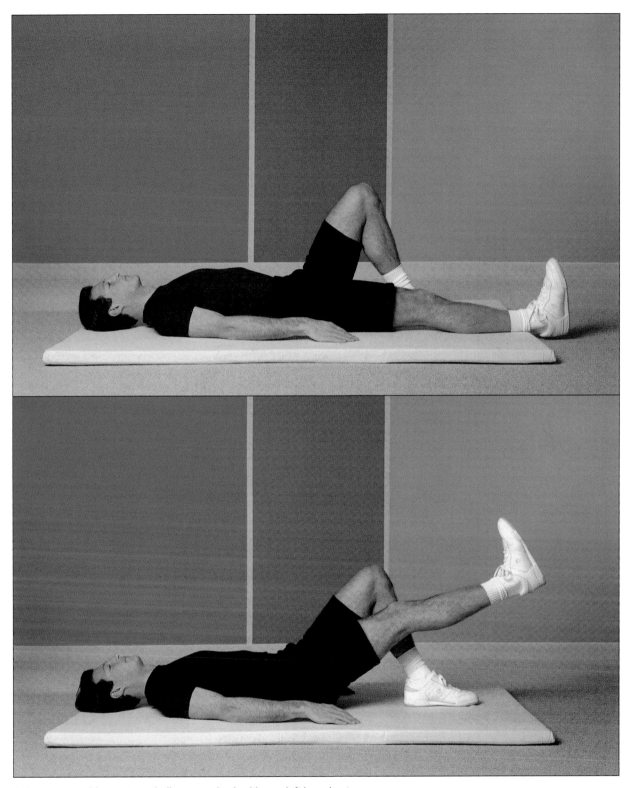

To increase quadriceps strength, lie on your back with your left knee bent and your left foot flat on the floor *(top)*. Raise your right leg about 30 centimetres or just until your back starts to arch *(above)*. Hold for 10 seconds; lower. Repeat this 15 times, then switch legs.

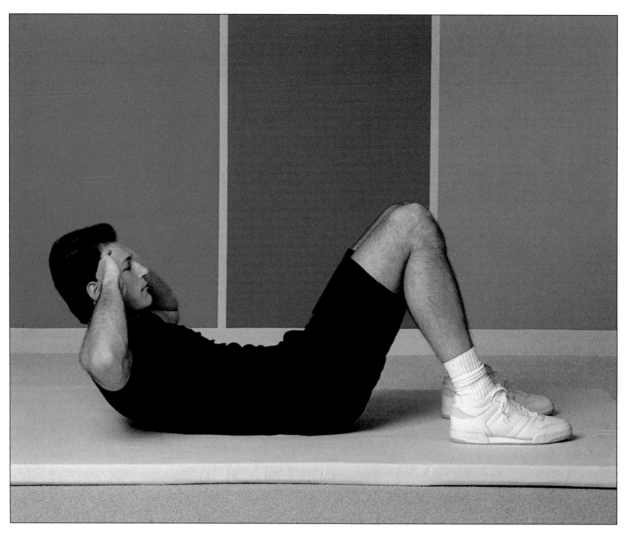

Advanced Strengtheners/1

To strengthen and tone your upper abdominals, lie on your back with your knees and elbows bent and your hands at your temples *(left)*. Raise your upper torso, keeping your arms open *(above)*. Perform three sets of 10 repetitions; work up to sets of 20 repetitions.

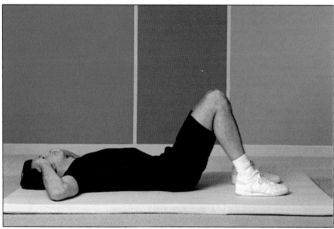

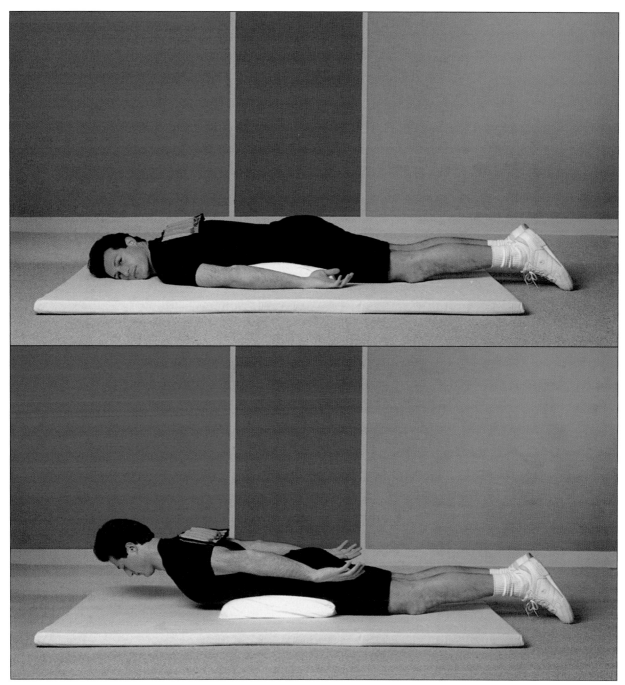

Place a 5-kilogram cuff weight across your upper back near your shoulders and lie face down with a pillow beneath your abdomen *(top)*. Raise your arms and upper torso *(above)*. Do three sets of 10 repetitions.

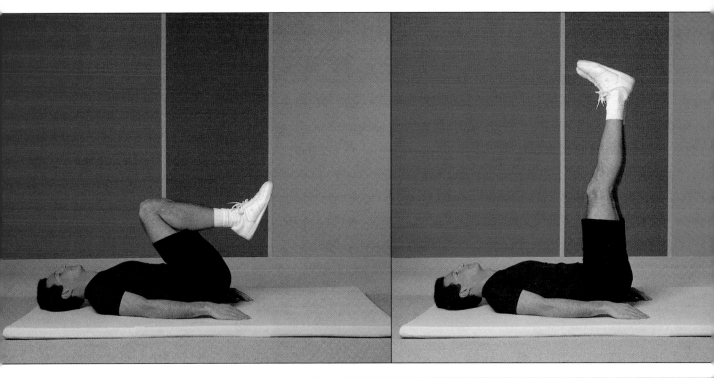

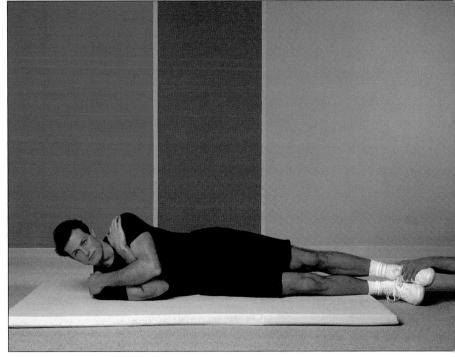

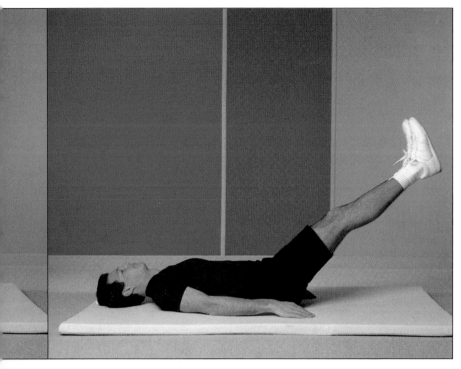

Advanced Strengtheners/2

Lie on your back with your arms at your sides. Bend your knees and lift your legs *(far left)*. Straighten your legs *(centre)*, then lower them together *(left)*. Stop lowering just before your lower back starts to arch. Use extreme caution to avoid arching your back. Return to the starting position. Beginning with one set of 10 repetitions, work up to two sets of 10 each.

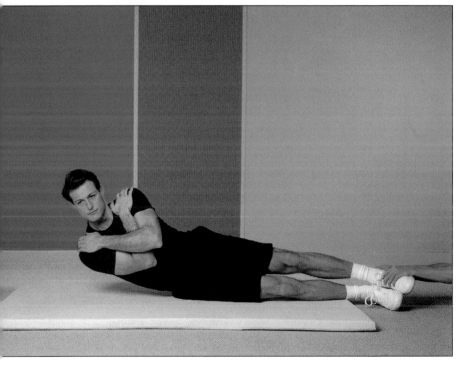

To strengthen both your abdominals and back muscles, lie on your right side and cross your arms in front of you so that your hands grasp your shoulders. Ask someone to hold your feet or hook them under a heavy piece of furniture *(far left)*. Raise your upper torso *(left)*. Hold momentarily; then lower. Start with five repetitions and work up to 10. Repeat on your left side.

Stretches/1

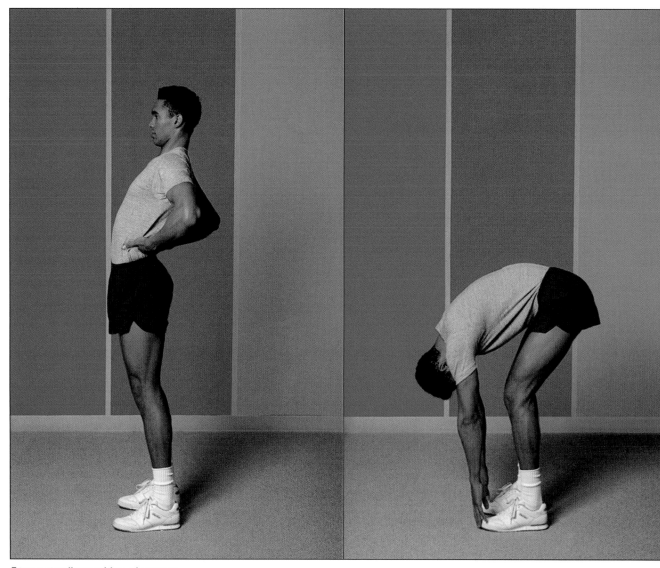

From a standing position, place your
hands behind your waist and draw your
shoulders together, arching your back
(above). Hold briefly, then drop your arms
to the floor and slowly bend forwards,
keeping your back rounded and bending
your knees slightly *(above, right)*. Perform
four full repetitions.

To stretch your chest muscles, stand
with your feet shoulder-width apart.
Grasp a rolled towel or stick behind your
back. Slowly raise your arms as far as
you can *(right)*. Hold, then lower.
Perform four repetitions.

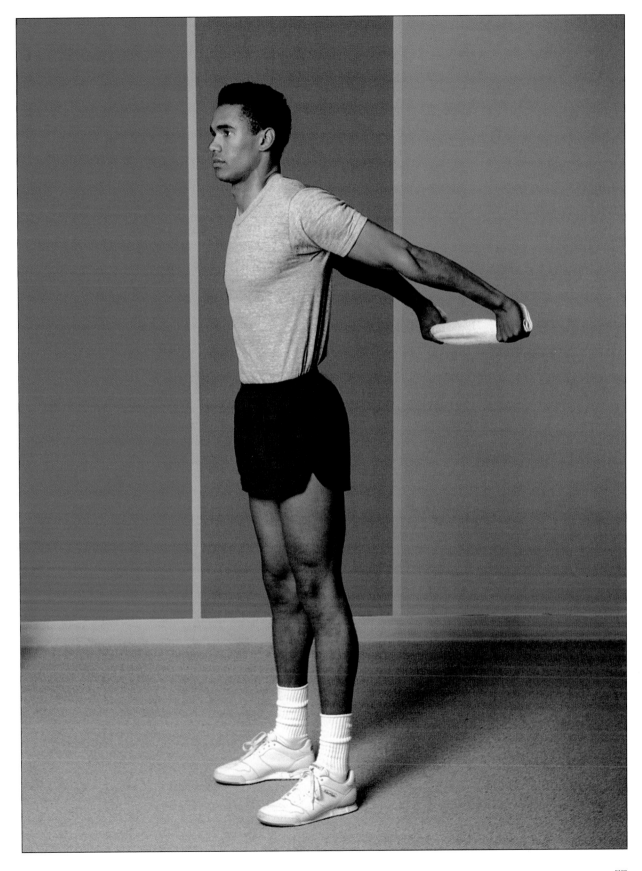

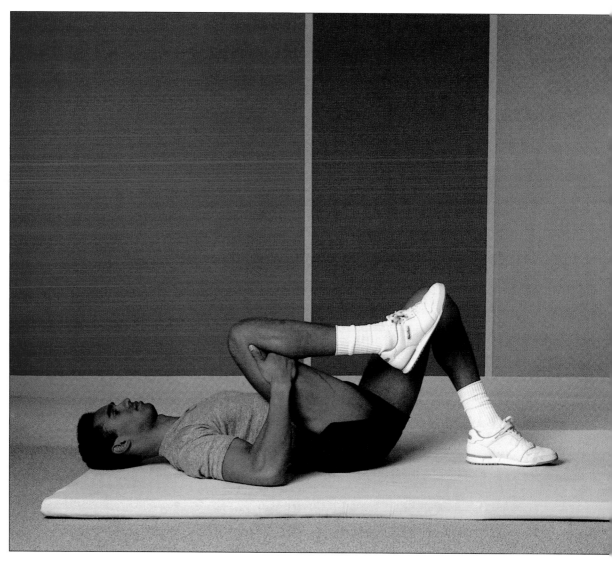

Stretches/2

Lie on your back with both knees bent.
Grasp your right thigh and pull your knee
to your chest *(above)*. Slowly straighten
your leg, keeping your foot relaxed
(opposite, above). Return to the second
position; perform four repetitions. Return
to the starting position and switch legs.

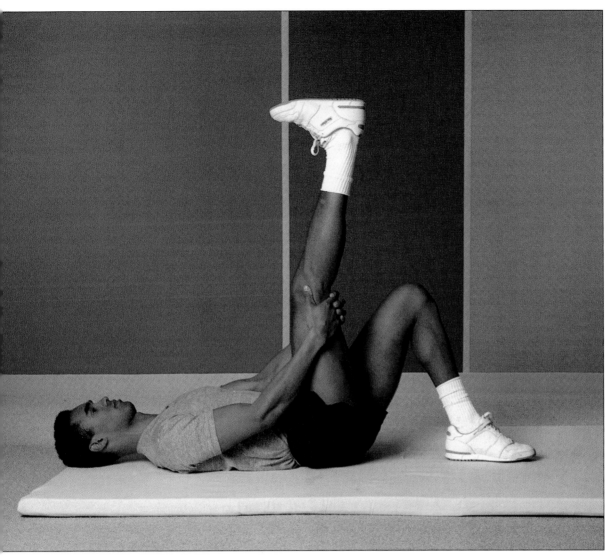

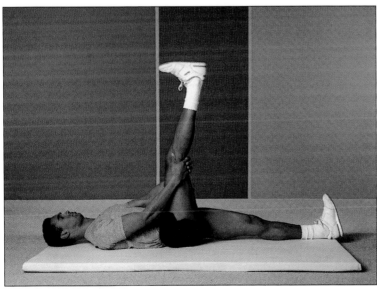

For a more difficult variation on the above exercise, keep your left leg straight when you lift the right, and vice versa.

Stretches/3

Stand at arm's length from a stool or table and extend your left leg behind you. Bend your right knee and, keeping your left leg straight, lean forwards, stretching your calf *(right)*. Hold for 10 seconds and relax. Perform four repetitions, then switch legs and repeat.

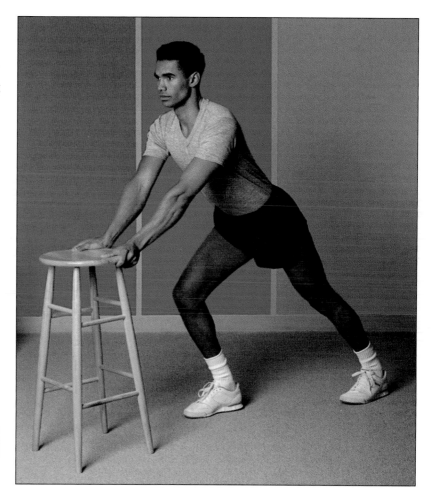

Lie on your abdomen with a pillow beneath you. Bend your left knee, bringing your foot backwards. Grasp it with your left hand and hold momentarily *(below)*. Perform four repetitions, then switch legs and repeat.

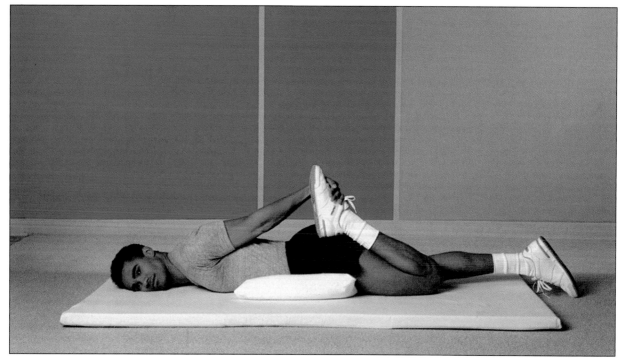

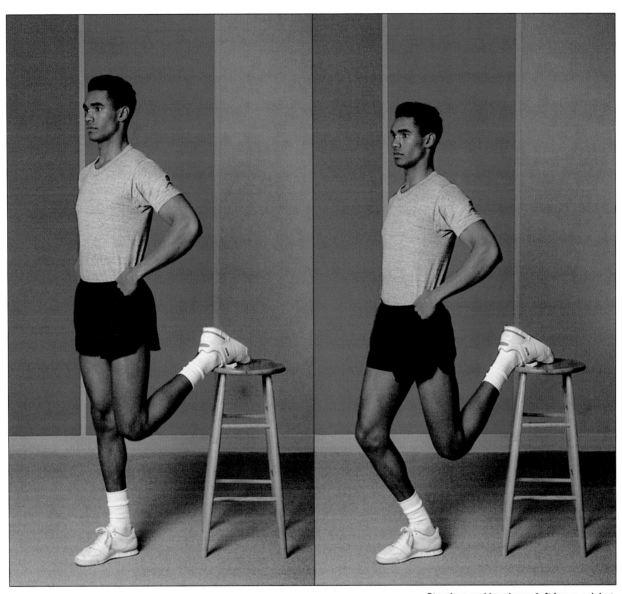

Stand up and bend your left knee, raising your foot and resting it behind you on a high stool or table *(above, left)*. Bend your right knee and lower your body *(above)*. Hold, keeping your back straight, then return to the starting position. Perform four repetitions, then switch legs.

Neck Stretches/1

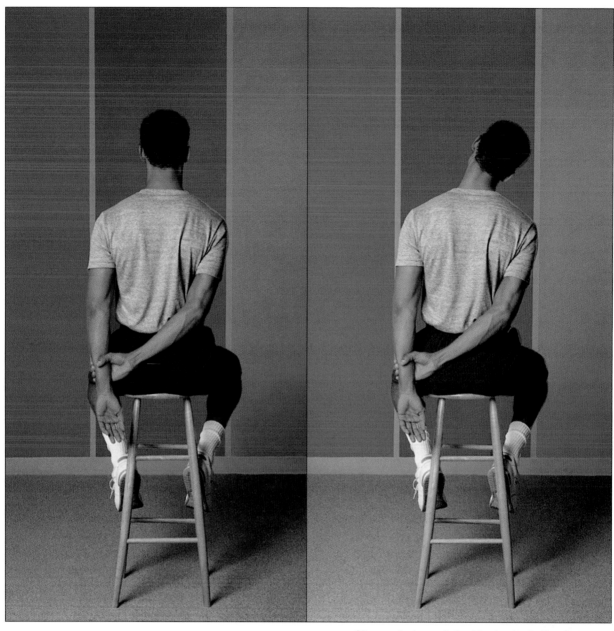

Sit on a stool or a chair with a low back. Keeping your left arm at your side, reach behind you and grasp your left arm just above the wrist with your right hand *(above, left)*. Simultaneously pull down on your left arm and lean your head to the right *(above)*. Return to the first position. Perform four repetitions, then switch arms and repeat.

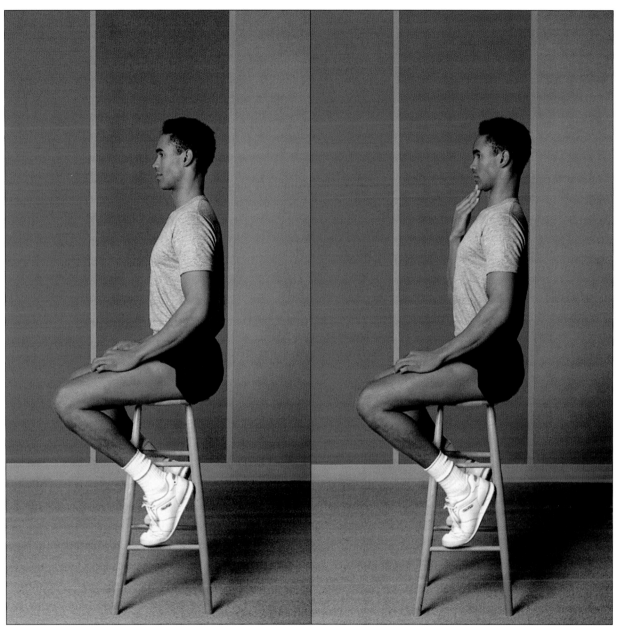

Look ahead as you sit straight on a stool or chair *(above, left)*. Slide your head backwards, keeping your gaze fixed. Raise your hand to your chin and press your chin inwards to increase the stretch to your neck muscles *(above)*. Hold this position momentarily; release. Perform four repetitions.

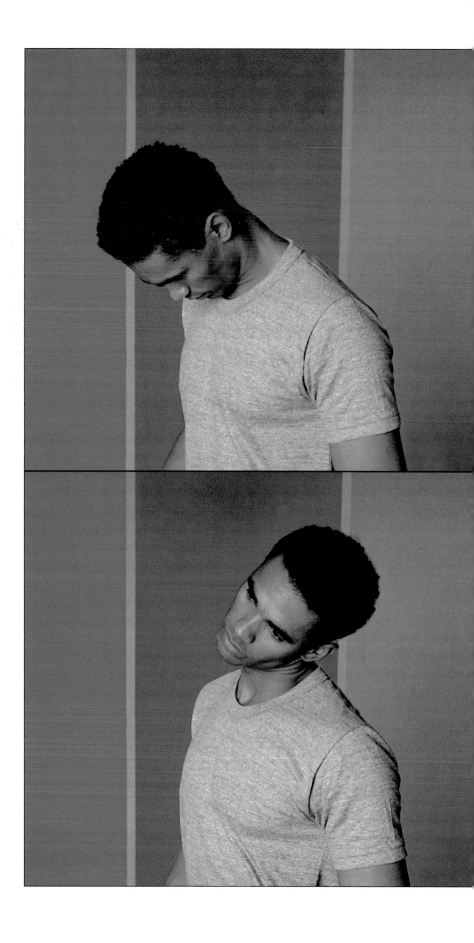

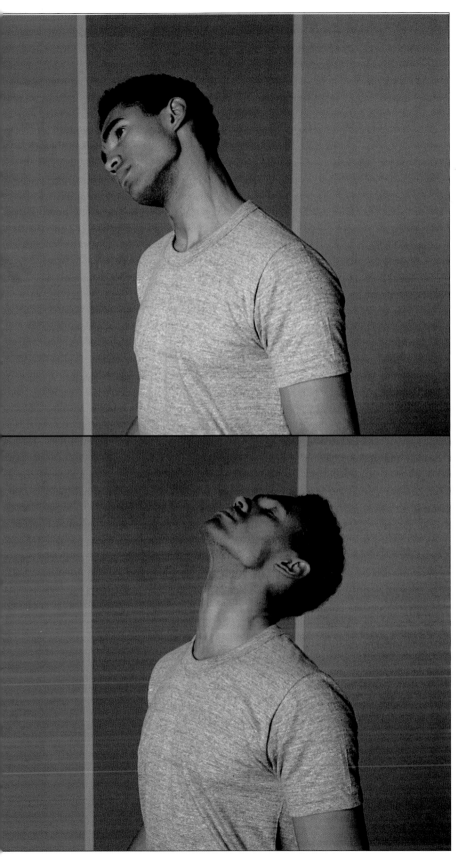

Neck Stretches/2

This exercise can be done from either a sitting or standing position. Clockwise from far left: drop your head to your chest; then slowly rotate it to your right; then backwards, taking care not to let your head drop back too abruptly; and finally to your left. Return to the starting position. Perform four repetitions.

Seated Stretches

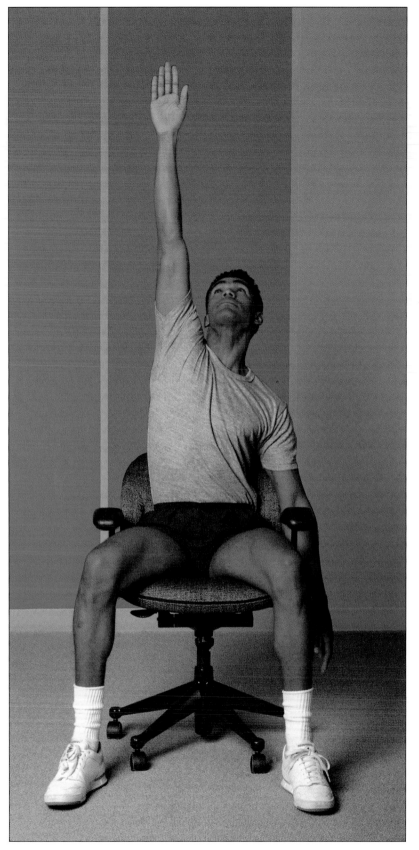

A good deal of the back strain that plagues many office workers develops from long hours of sitting. With prolonged sitting, the back extensor muscles that allow the back to bend become either lengthened or shortened. If you have a desk job, it is imperative to maintain back mobility by standing and walking at frequent intervals during the day.

Additionally, you can perform some stretches sitting at your desk to maintain joint mobility and to retain muscle flexibility. The exercises on these two pages mimic some of the standing stretches on the previous pages, but they are modified for sitting. They stretch not only the neck muscles but the muscles of both the upper and lower back. Because these exercises take a minimum of time and effort, they can be performed several times throughout the day.

Sit with your back against the back of your chair. Reach straight up from your shoulder with your right arm, looking upwards to extend the stretch through your side. Hold then lower and switch arms. Perform four repetitions.

To increase back mobility, sit with your back firmly against the back of your chair. Clockwise from top left: place your hands on the back of your chair and stretch backwards, then drop your hands to the floor and lean forwards with your head between your knees. Come back up and place your hands behind your waist, arching your back forwards, then grasp the arm or side of the chair and turn to the left; switch sides and turn to your right. Perform four repetitions.

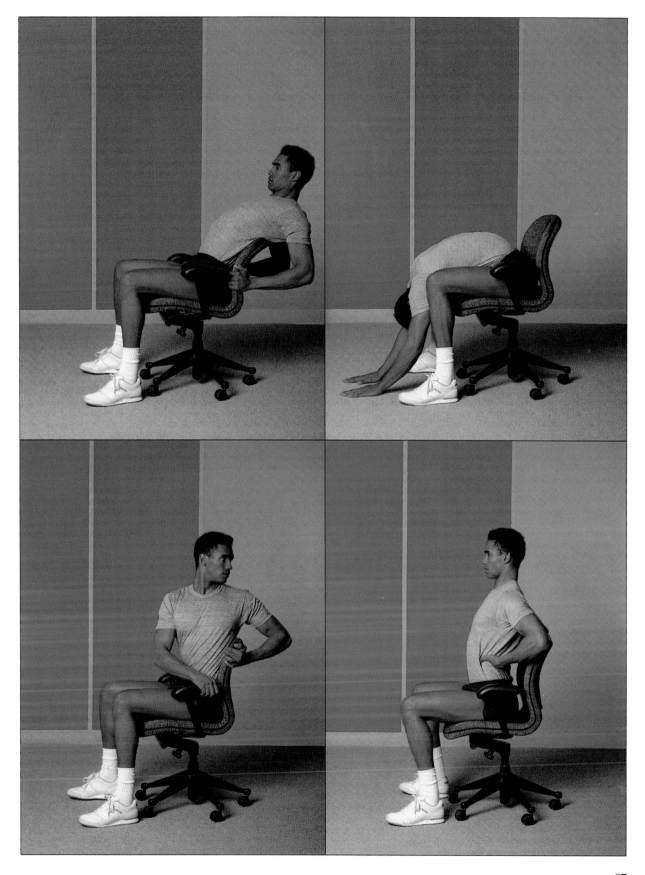

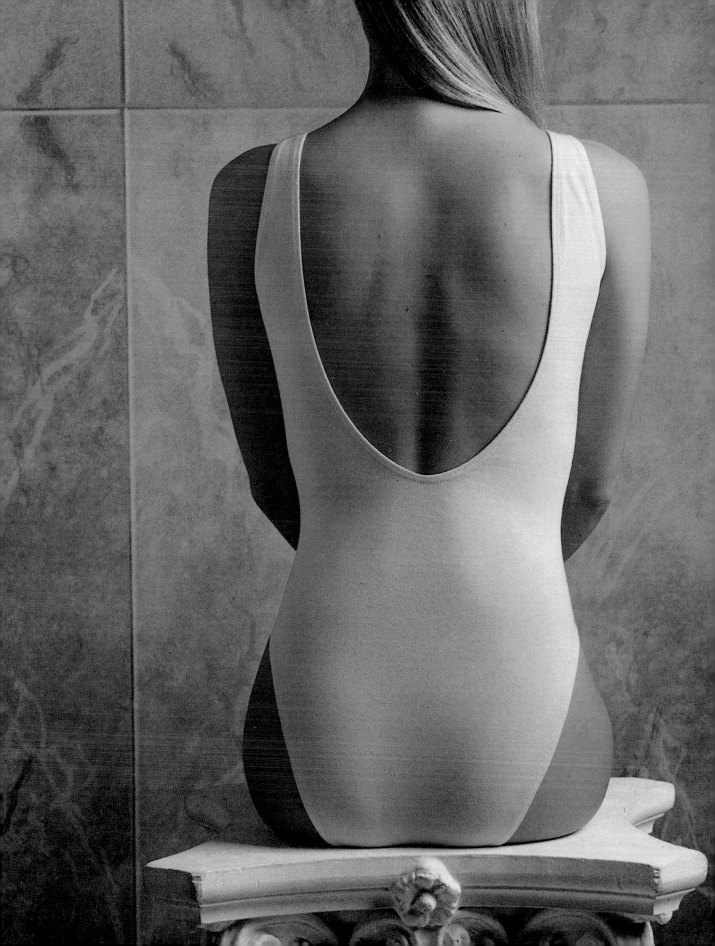

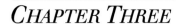

CHAPTER THREE

Posture

*For minimal back stress
and maximum ease of
movement*

Ｉt is frequently assumed — wrongly — that to have proper posture you should mimic the traditional military attention stance characterized by pulled-back shoulders, tucked-in chin and excessively arched lower back. Unlike this static, rigid configuration, posture is dynamic, and so requires continual adjustments. It incorporates the countless ways in which you align your spine and its supporting structures to allow common everyday positions such as sitting, standing, sleeping and carrying.

Good posture — keeping your spine aligned in a correct and comfortable position — demands careful balancing among the many bones, joints and muscles of the back. When the back is properly aligned, you will maximize the spaces between the 24 vertebrae along the spinal column, thus lengthening the spine and allowing the vertebrae to move easily in relation to one another. The advantage of this maximum spacing is that it avoids spinal compression, thus placing the least possible stress on your spine. Correct posture also allows you to maintain the desired configuration of the three curves in your back: the forward curves of the neck and lower back, and the backward curve of the middle spine.

Poor posture often leads to an exaggeration of the back's normal curves. In particular, sway-back — a hyperlordosis, or excessive curvature, of the lower back — contributes significantly to back problems by pulling the vertebrae of the lower back out of alignment. The misalignment compresses the facet joints at the back of the vertebrae, causing them to wear down. Abnormal spinal alignment also places demands on the supporting ligaments and musculature of the back, forcing certain muscles to compensate, while others are underutilized.

Not only is posture dynamic, it is interdependent, involving the head, shoulders, hips and legs as well as the spine itself. For example, an exaggerated curvature in one area of the back can lead to compensating misalignments elsewhere. Thus, if you have sway-back, you might very well have hyperkyphosis, or a rounded upper back and shoulders, plus hyperlordosis in the neck. Similarly, incorrect lifting — using the back muscles rather than the quadriceps muscles in the thighs — can strain the back extensors, thus reducing their effectiveness in spinal support. Because of this interdependence, many back-care specialists nowadays tend to treat the whole body, including the neck, shoulders and hip joints.

There is a reciprocal relationship between posture and the supporting musculature of the back: good muscle tone is necessary for proper posture, and proper posture enables your muscles to function appropriately. For example, strong abdominal muscles will allow you to maintain the optimum curve in your lower back, while weak abdominals permit the spine to curve forwards, creating a hyperlordosis, which shortens the muscles of the back and compresses the vertebrae.

Improving the tone of the muscles that support your spine will help to reduce excess curvatures. However, good muscle tone does not in itself necessarily guarantee good posture. Even if your overall muscle tone is quite adequate, poor habits such as slumped sitting, stooped standing and rounded shoulders can develop over a period of years, frequently beginning in adolescence.

Retraining yourself to overcome bad posture can be a challenge. Because they are familiar, the positions you commonly assume for standing and sitting probably feel right to you. Therefore, edicts such as "sit up straight", or "pull your head back" are likely to elicit a temporary response at best. Some researchers believe that performing exercises aimed at improving your sense of what feels correct is the most effective approach to undoing bad habits.

The Alexander technique is one method that uses self-awareness to "teach" the entire spine and back to move with less stress and greater efficiency. Developed at the turn of the century by F.M. Alexander, the technique helps you replace dysfunctional movement habits with improved ones. In one study based on the Alexander technique,

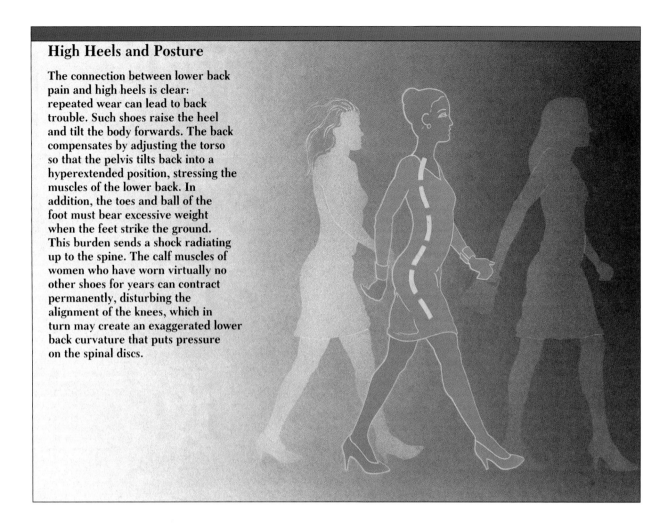

High Heels and Posture

The connection between lower back pain and high heels is clear: repeated wear can lead to back trouble. Such shoes raise the heel and tilt the body forwards. The back compensates by adjusting the torso so that the pelvis tilts back into a hyperextended position, stressing the muscles of the lower back. In addition, the toes and ball of the foot must bear excessive weight when the feet strike the ground. This burden sends a shock radiating up to the spine. The calf muscles of women who have worn virtually no other shoes for years can contract permanently, disturbing the alignment of the knees, which in turn may create an exaggerated lower back curvature that puts pressure on the spinal discs.

participants were first told to sit in their normal relaxed position. They were then told to correct their sitting in two ways: first by simply being directed to sit up straight and second by being guided into an improved sitting alignment using Alexander principles. Neck muscle tension of participants increased sharply when they were merely told to sit up straight, but they experienced a marked decrease in muscular tension — coupled with the desired spine lengthening — when they used the Alexander instructions.

The Alexander-based exercises in this chapter are designed to train muscles during ordinary movement so that you will become familiar with good posture as you sit, stand and walk. Some exercises, such as those in the sitting alignment routine on pages 80-81, demonstrate the different sensations that good and bad posture create. Others, such as the shoulder circles on page 86, tone the muscles associated with posture as they improve alignment. As you become increasingly familiar with how your back feels when you move through these positions, you will find it relatively easy to discard your old postural habits and replace them with improved ones.

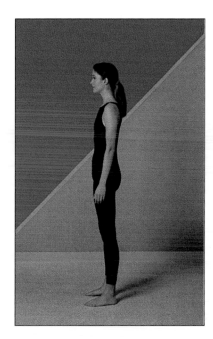

Standing/1

Stand with your feet spread slightly and your arms at your sides *(above)*. Tighten your abdominals as you raise your arms over your head in front of you *(right)*. Keep your arms shoulder-width apart. Return to the starting position. Do four repetitions.

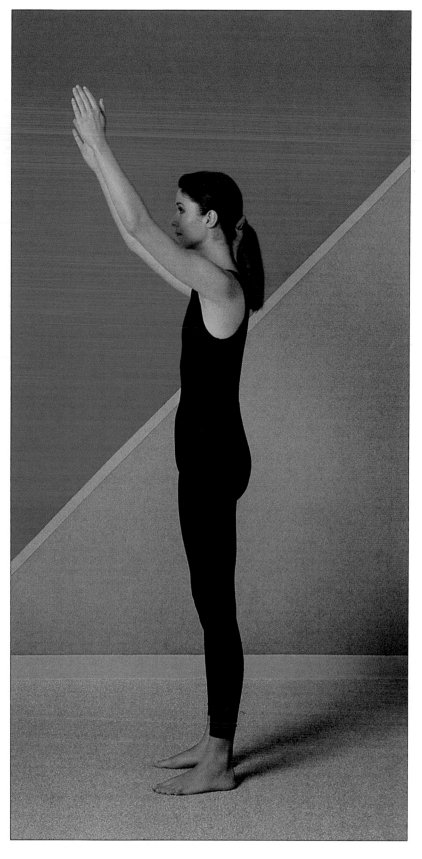

Aligning Your Spine

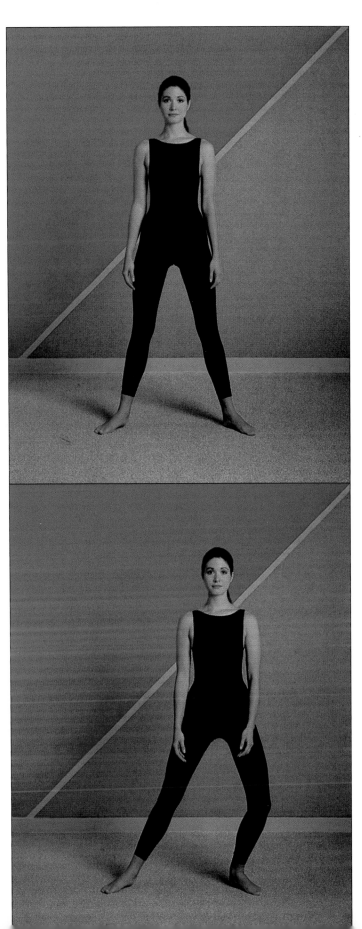

The basic principle behind the exercises on these two pages and the following 18 pages is to keep your spine aligned and elongated, achieving the maximum possible length from your neck to your coccyx. To visualize this while you perform the exercises, imagine a thread being pulled gently from the top of your head, drawing your spine upwards as it positions the vertebrae on top of one another.

The exercises are not designed to be strenuous, but rather to encourage postural awareness and help you acquire habits that you can use in everyday activities. Thus, careful monitoring of your movements and exacting adjustments are far more important than the speed of the execution or the number of repetitions. If possible, perform the exercises in front of a mirror so that you can observe the curvatures of your spine.

Practise the exercises daily. Doing so while imagining your spine in proper alignment will retrain your posture habits. Through the process of exercise combined with picturing your spine and observation, you can internalize new ways of moving so that you can go through your daily activities with grace and efficiency.

Take a comfortably wide stance with your arms at your sides *(top)*. **Bend your left knee, letting your torso move to the left. Keep your spine lengthened** *(left)*. **Straighten your knee; repeat to the right. Alternate sides 10 times.**

Standing/2

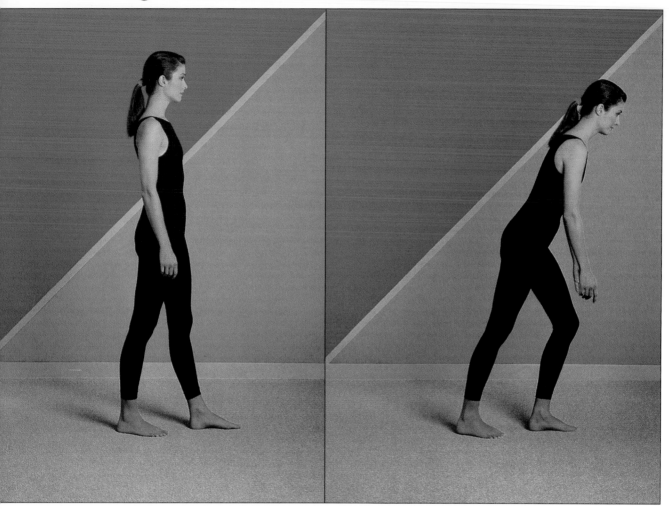

Stand straight with your feet slightly spread and your left foot in front of your right *(above)*. Lean forwards, bending your left knee and keeping your back straight *(above, right)*. Straighten your leg and return to the starting position. Repeat the movement five times, then switch legs.

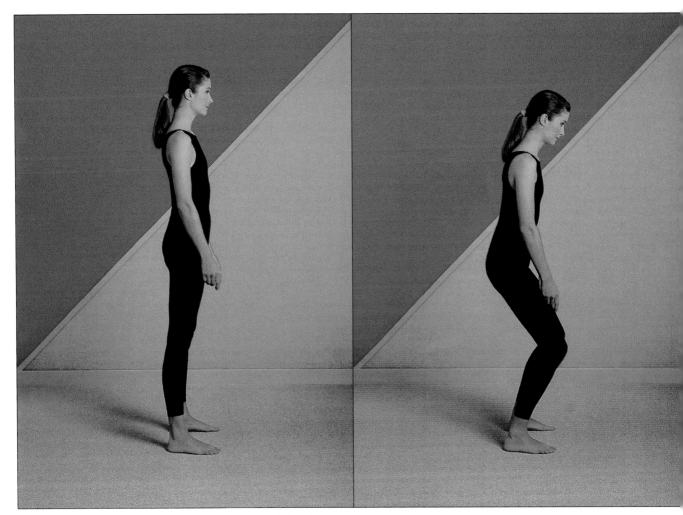

Stand straight with your feet shoulder-width apart *(above)*, bend both knees and lean forwards *(above, right)*. Keep your spine aligned and use your hips to tilt your torso forwards. Keep your arms relaxed; straighten your body. Repeat five times.

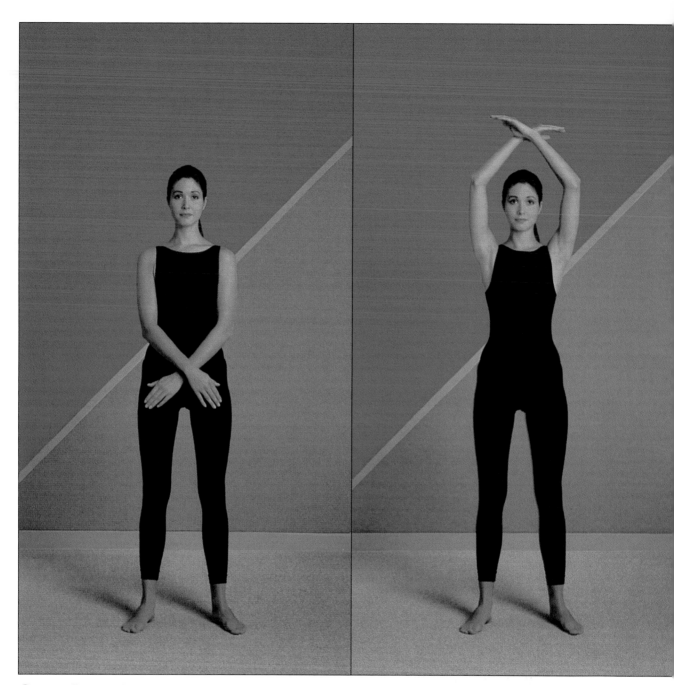

Standing/3

Stand with your feet shoulder-width apart and cross your arms
in front of you *(above)*. Make large arm circles by slowly raising
your crossed arms *(above, right)*, then opening them up *(opposite,
left)* and bringing them down to your sides *(opposite, right)*.
Return to the starting position and repeat five times.

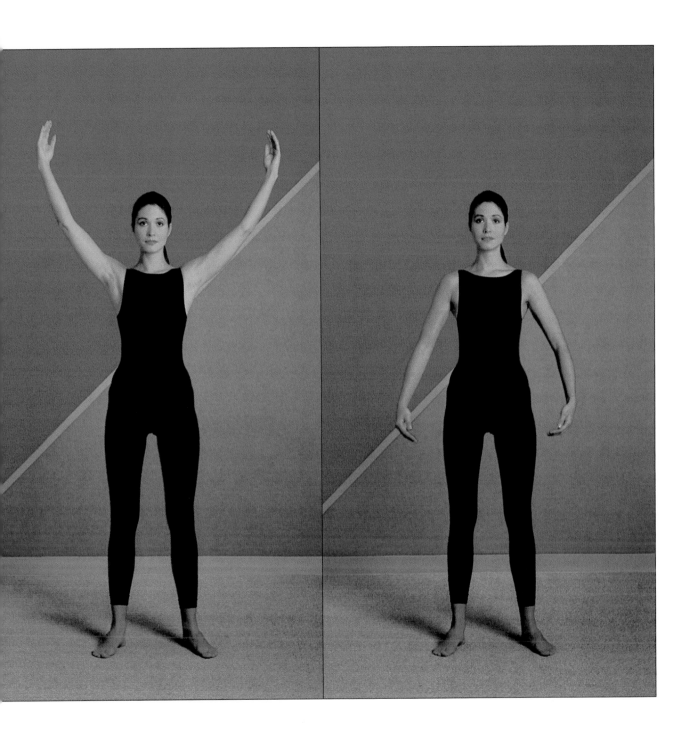

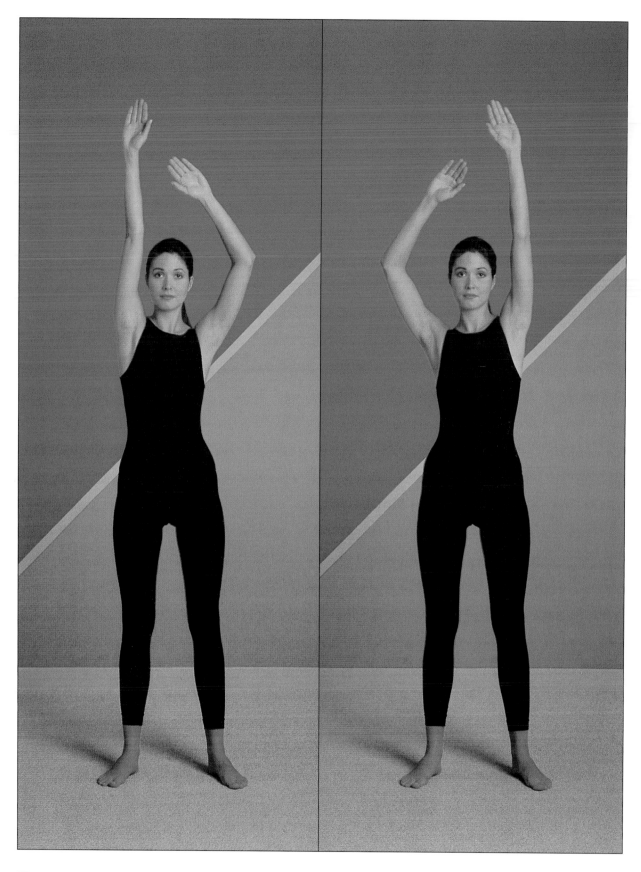

Standing/4

Raise your arms over your head, keeping
them shoulder-width apart. Alternately
reach up with your right and then your left
arm *(opposite)*. Tighten your abdominals
as you reach. Alternate arms 10 times.

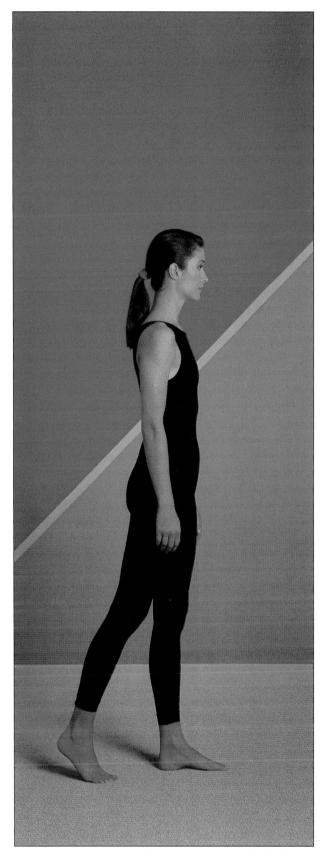

Walk for one minute, keeping your spine
lengthened and your arms relaxed at your
sides. Alternate tightening your
abdominals for four steps and releasing
them for the next four steps.

79

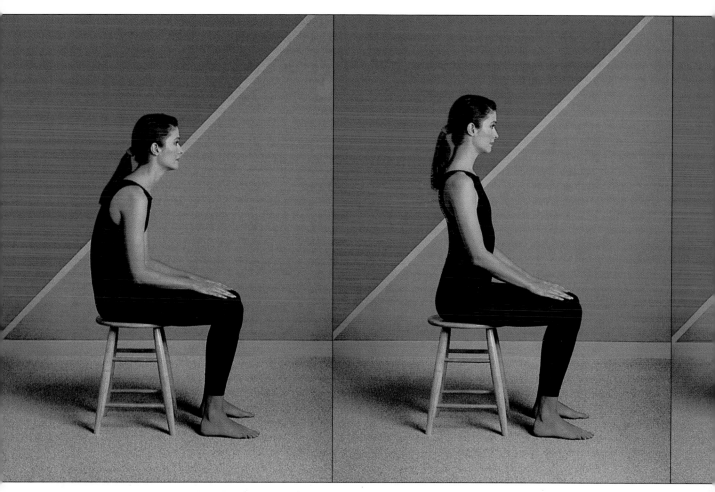

Sitting/1

Sit on a stool or a chair with your back unsupported. To find your correct body alignment, slouch forwards *(above)*, then arch your lower back as much as possible *(above, centre)*, then assume an upright position between these two extremes *(above, right)*. Repeat three times.

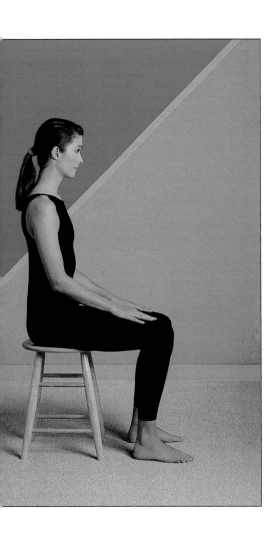

Place one hand loosely round the back of your neck. While looking straight ahead, gently bring your neck back towards your hand as you think of lengthening your neck and entire spine. Hold for a count of five; repeat the exercise three times.

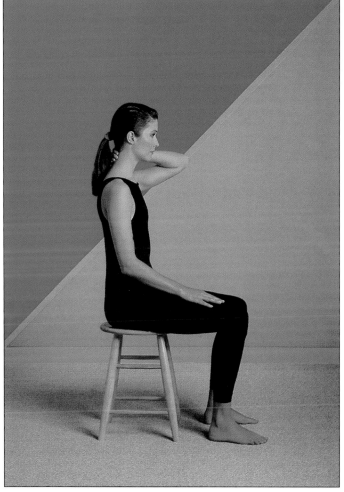

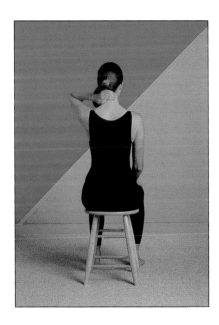

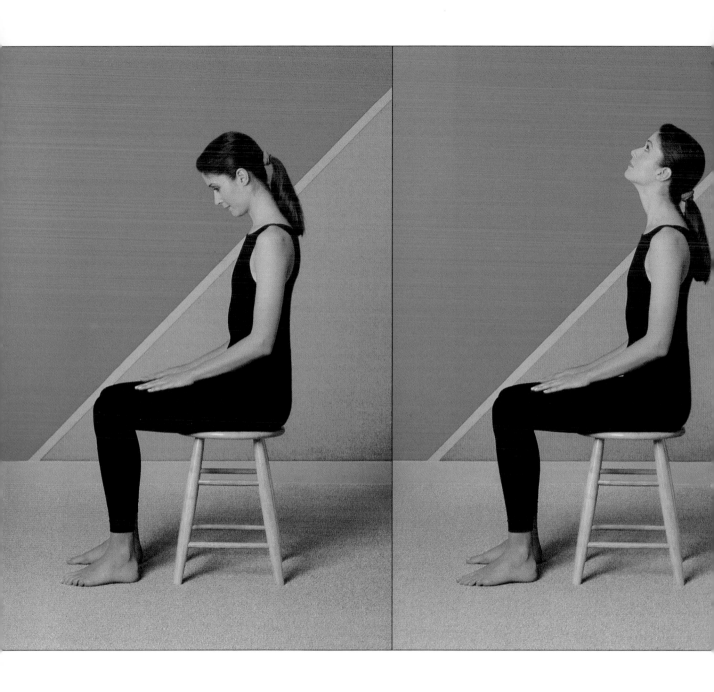

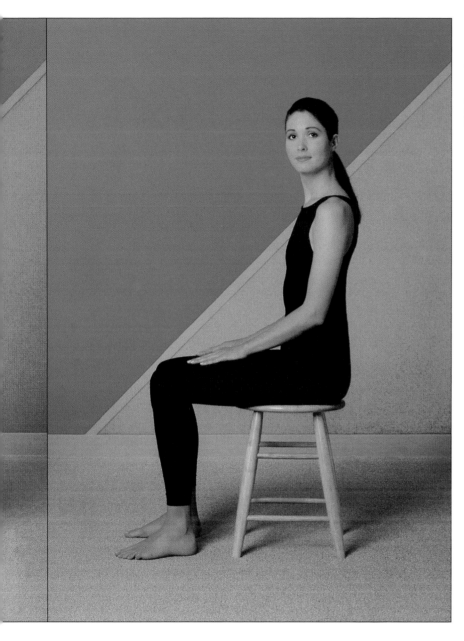

Sitting/2

Sit on a chair or stool with your feet flat on the floor, your hands resting on your lap and your back straight. Look down *(far left)*, look up *(centre)*, then look to each side *(left)*. Make sure you keep your spine lengthened as you move your head. Repeat five times.

Sitting/3

Clockwise from top left: sit on a stool
with your hands at your sides. Raise your
arms and extend them out to the sides,
keeping your shoulders even. Raise your
arms over your head and bend your
elbows so that your forearms rest lightly
on your head. Raise your arms back up,
out and down to return to the starting
position, as you lengthen your head and
spine. Repeat three times.

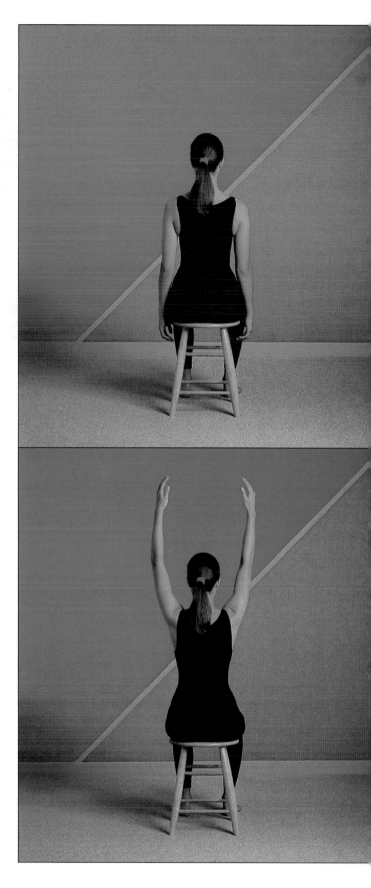

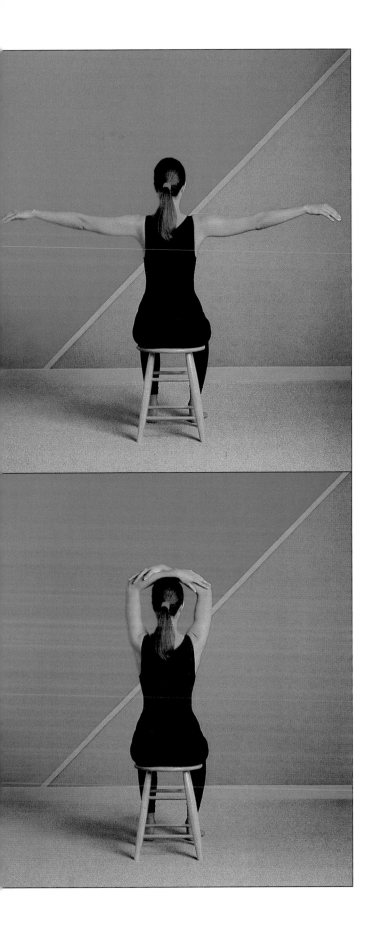

Sitting/4

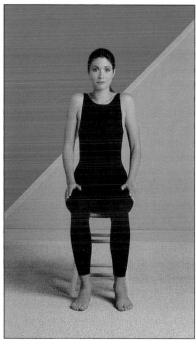

From a sitting position, circle your shoulders by bringing them up *(above)*, back *(right)*, down and forwards. Keep your spine lengthened. Repeat five times.

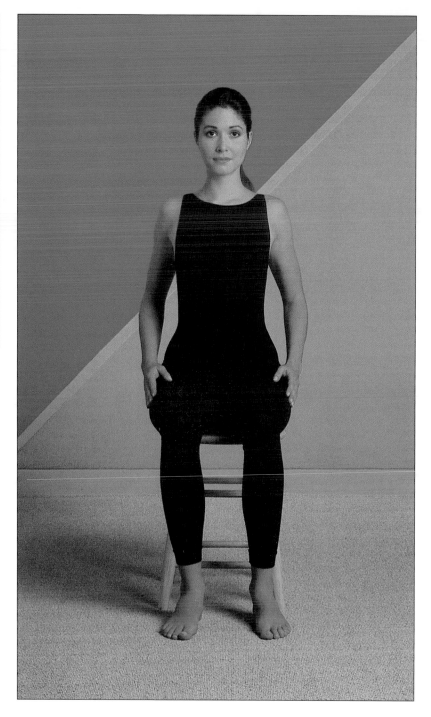

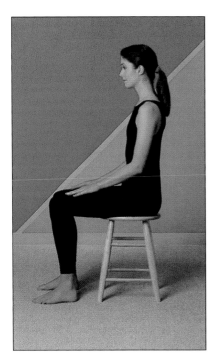

Sit on a chair or stool with your spine
lengthened and your feet flat on the floor
in front of you *(above)*. Lean forwards
keeping your spine aligned *(right)*. Return
to the starting position. Repeat five times.

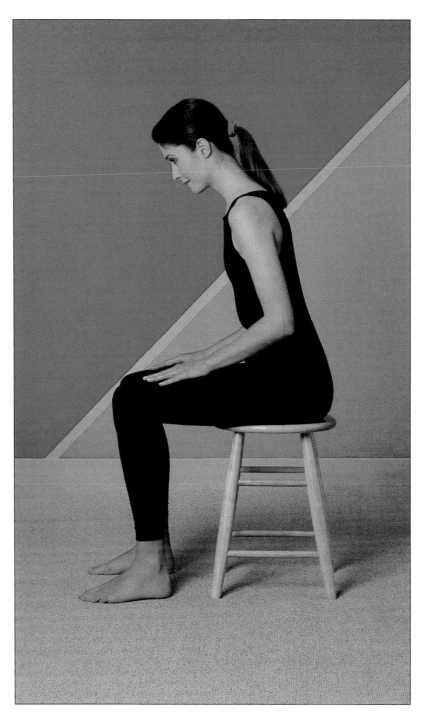

Sitting/5

Sit erect on a chair or stool with your
spine elongated and your hands resting
lightly on your thighs. Gently tighten your
abdominals five times.

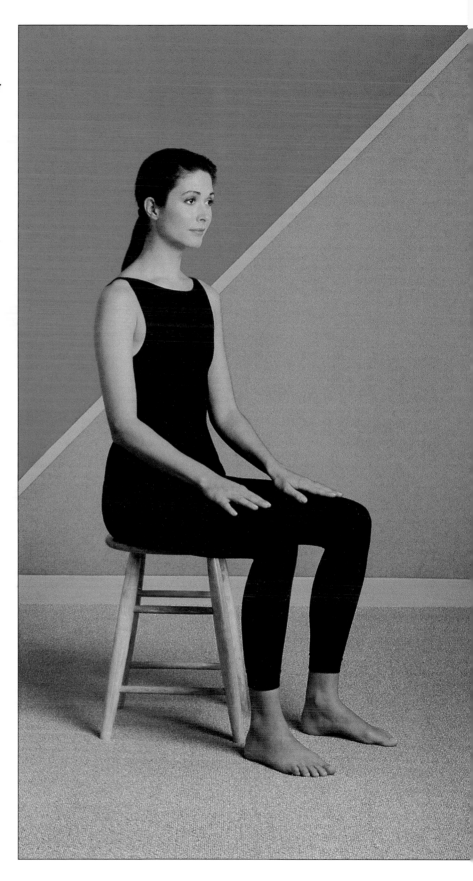

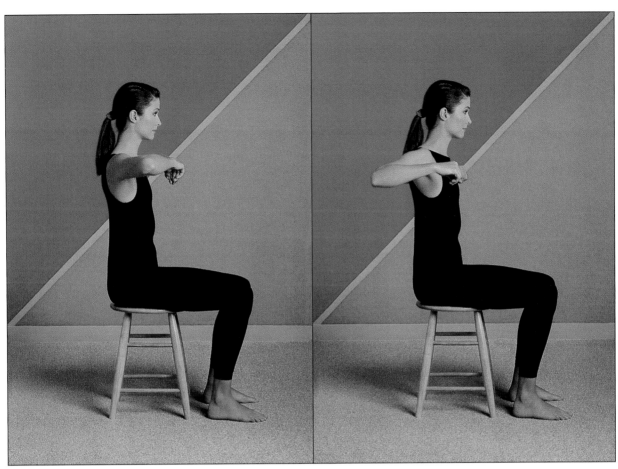

While seated, raise your arms out to the side to shoulder height, with your elbows bent *(above, left)*. Pull your shoulders back five times, drawing your shoulder blades together *(above)*; lower your arms. Repeat three times.

Lying Down

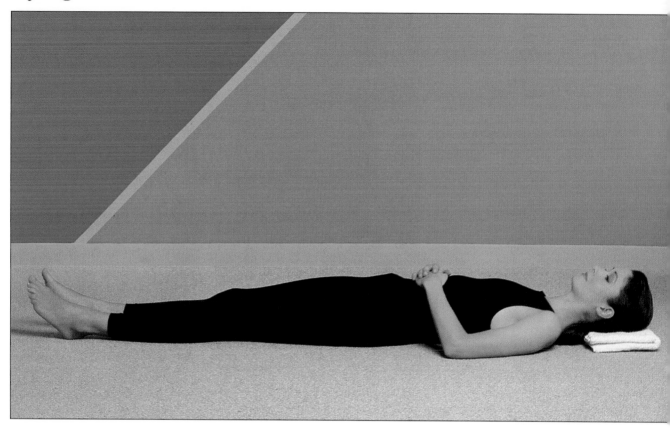

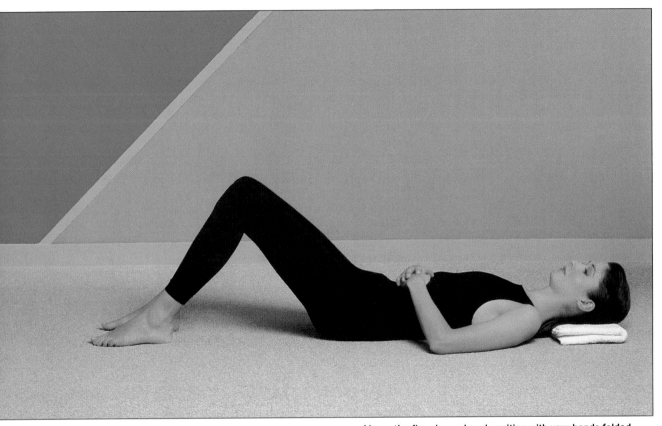

Lie on the floor in a relaxed position with your hands folded over your abdomen *(opposite)*. Place a small pillow or folded towel under your head to keep your neck aligned. Bend your legs so that your feet lie flat on the floor *(above)*. Keeping your hips in place, stretch your spine by flattening your lower back against the floor, and then moving your shoulders and head along the floor away from your hips. Maintaining this alignment, rest for a count of 10 or longer.

Breathing Techniques

All of the back muscles that attach to the ribs or that lie below them are affected by breathing. Correct breathing enables this musculature to relax and keeps it well supplied with oxygen. Indeed, breathing correctly helps to promote relaxation and can even reduce back problems by breaking the cycle of tension and pain.

Improving your posture by performing exercises such as those shown on the preceding 20 pages can ease your breathing. When you reduce spinal compression, you provide more room for your muscles to expand and contract freely. This is particularly important for the diaphragm, the primary muscle involved in breathing. This muscle is attached to the lower ribs as well as to some of the vertebrae of the spine. Overtightening the muscles of the chest and neck will interfere with correct breathing. In contrast, a well-balanced spine allows you to use your diaphragm and other muscles to breathe correctly.

You can tell if you are breathing properly by the way your abdomen and rib cage move: on inhalation, they should expand, and on exhalation, they move back inwards. The two exercises shown here will help you evaluate your breathing and concentrate on improving it.

Sit up straight in a chair. Place your hands on either side of your rib cage, with your thumbs towards your back. Breathe naturally. Keep your spine lengthened as you feel your ribs move in and out with each breath.

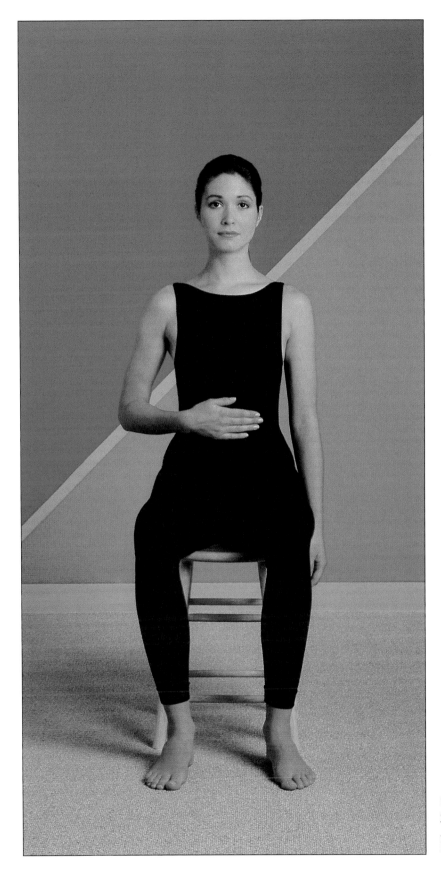

Place one hand at the centre of your abdomen at waist level. Breathe naturally. You should feel your abdomen expand as you breathe in and move inwards as you breathe out.

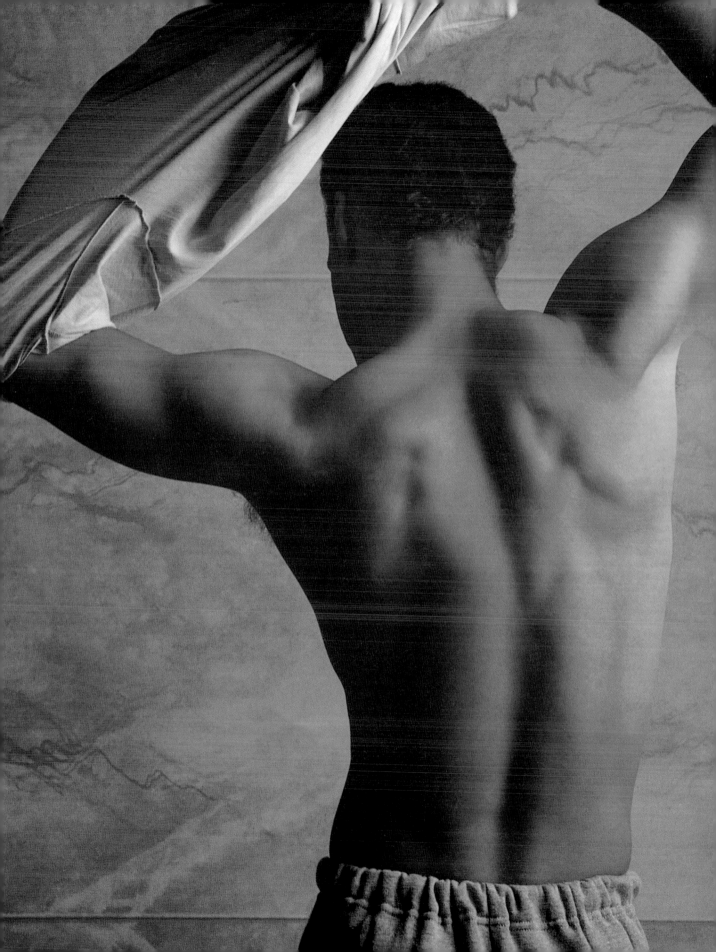

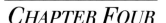
Day-to-Day Back Care

Techniques for protecting your back in everyday situations

G ood posture and well-toned muscles provide the foundation for a fit back, but these two basic elements of back care are effective only if you ensure that you integrate them into the performance of simple daily activities such as driving a car, lifting an infant, carrying a suitcase and other similar manoeuvres that can become sources of back strain. This chapter will show you efficient ways of standing, sitting and moving that you can apply to almost any situation that involves your back.

The spine's flexibility allows you to combine considerable mobility with strength. When done properly, any normal movement is within the spine's range and can be performed without any strain. Unfortunately, the spine is often used incorrectly. In particular, the waist is commonly used as a hinge joint between the lower and the upper body, forcing it to work like a knee or an elbow. But the waist is not a joint, and trying to use it as one can strain or overstretch the muscles and ligaments of the lower back.

For bending movements, the hips allow the torso — pelvis and spine — to move forwards as a unit. Actions such as bending, leaning and lifting should all be accomplished with the hips rather than the waist. This will allow you to use the muscles of the torso correctly to maintain vertebral alignment.

Lifting offers one of the best examples of the importance of moving properly. No other common manoeuvre places as much stress on the lower back as picking up an object from the floor with your knees straight and your torso bent at the waist. The bent-knee technique, which is demonstrated on pages 104-105, illustrates the correct way to lift: flexing your hips and bending your knees, using the quadriceps muscles in the front of the thigh for power and concentrating on upper body alignment. Your abdominals and the large muscles of the thigh share the burden of lowering and lifting, relieving the back muscles and the spine itself of the load.

Another common activity that poses risks to the lower back is sitting. In fact, sitting creates more strain than walking, standing or lying down, and its stresses account largely for the high incidence of lower back pain among office workers. Doctors report that many years spent sitting in office jobs can cause a condition known as fibrous contracture, characterized by a shortening of the muscles in the back and a resulting loss of elasticity. This condition of overall inflexibility often makes it difficult and even painful for the sufferer to bend forwards.

One of the best ways to ease the stress of sitting is to find a good chair. A soft, overstuffed sofa can be just as hard on the back as a backless stool or poorly designed desk chair — none of them provides adequate lower back support. When you choose a chair, find one with a firm, padded, adjustable back that can tilt backwards about 10 degrees. Its seat should support your thighs at a 90-degree angle to your lower legs, or your knees can be slightly higher than your hips. If you do not have a suitable chair, maintaining proper posture and using cushions for lumbar support can still help overcome the strain of prolonged sitting *(see pages 108-109)*. Interrupting periods of sitting with stretching, walking or simply shifting positions is recommended to prevent your back from becoming stiff and inflexible. Examples of good chairs, lumbar pillows and other items that are designed for the back are given on pages 98-99.

Some people react to potential back problems by overprotecting themselves and avoiding activities — including sports and sex — that they fear might trigger back pain. In fact, physical activity can actually benefit the back, as long as the activity is carefully chosen *(see box, opposite)*. You do not have to forego sex unless you have acute back pain and muscle spasm; otherwise, you need only take care to use positions for intercourse that are easy on your back. Many back specialists recommend lying on your side, either facing your partner or lying back to front. Alternatively, if the partner with the back problem is on top during sex, he or she will be more comfortable if the other

Choosing a Sport

Having a back problem is one reason to avoid sports, but you should follow certain guidelines in deciding which sport or exercise routines to engage in. The most important rule is to maintain proper conditioning of the back's supporting muscles. Strong, flexible muscles are the best guarantee of staying injury-free. Here are other tips to keep in mind:

◆ The exercises most highly recommended for people with back problems are swimming (except for the butterfly and breaststroke, in which you must arch your back), walking, cross-country skiing and cycling (as long as you use an upright posture). These particular sports are also excellent cardiovascular conditioners, so that you will build endurance as you improve your back muscles.

◆ In the poorly conditioned individual, racket sports, golf and other activities that involve twisting the torso can imperil the back. Bowling can also pose a risk because it involves lifting a heavy weight. Besides straining the back muscles, a sudden twist can cause a ruptured disc if the movement is too abrupt. Sports-medicine specialists have noted, however, that such injuries tend to occur because of incorrect techniques or insufficient warm-ups, not because they are intrinsic to any sport.

◆ Certain other exercise movements can put you at risk of back pain. Running and aerobic dance can be jarring to the back, but you can minimize the stress by wearing proper shoes and working out on a surface resilient enough to cushion the shock. If you are performing routines to improve muscle tone, be sure to avoid straight-leg sit-ups and bilateral leg-lifts, which can irritate the spinal nerves. If you lift weights, take care not to overarch your back. It is also wise to wear a lifting belt and to work with a spotter.

person is propped up with a couple of extra cushions. This facilitates a bent-knee position for the partner on top, because it tilts the pelvis forwards to minimize lower back stress.

The techniques that are described in the following 18 pages will help you put into practice the postural and muscular development outlined in the previous chapters. Indeed, the practical movement applications demonstrated in this chapter are really extensions of the preceding routines. Understanding these concepts and retraining your body to these new ways of moving will go a long way towards helping you to maintain a healthy back.

The chapter concludes with trigger point and massage sequences that you and your partner can use. Both trigger point and massage therapy are commonly used in the physical rehabilitation of back patients. However, they serve important preventive functions as well. In its most basic form, trigger point therapy entails a simple finger-pressure technique that can pinpoint and alleviate specific problems that may contribute to back pain. Likewise, massage is a hands-on therapy that eases overall muscle tension in your back. Using both of these techniques as a regular part of your back-care regimen is a pleasant and relaxing way to protect your back from the strain that it can undergo during the course of a day.

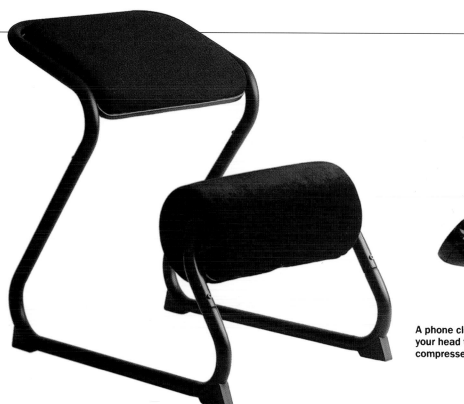

A kneeling chair, by putting the weight of your body on your knees, encourages your torso to maintain balance and alignment.

A phone clip prevents you from tilting your head to your shoulder, which compresses your cervical spine.

Lumbar cushions can provide the lower back support that a chair, couch or car seat may lack.

Back Aids

Having the proper equipment and furniture can facilitate back care, as well as prevent back pain or injury. There is no dearth of products designed to benefit your back; however, all such items are user-specific. Because what is comfortable for someone else might be irritating to your back, it is important to try out anything you intend to purchase, particularly chairs and mattresses. Similarly, although back-supporting equipment and furniture comes in a wide range of prices, cost is not necessarily a true indicator of either quality or appropriateness for an individual.

A sampling of chairs and accessories intended to provide maximum support and to relieve muscular tension in the back area appears on these two pages.

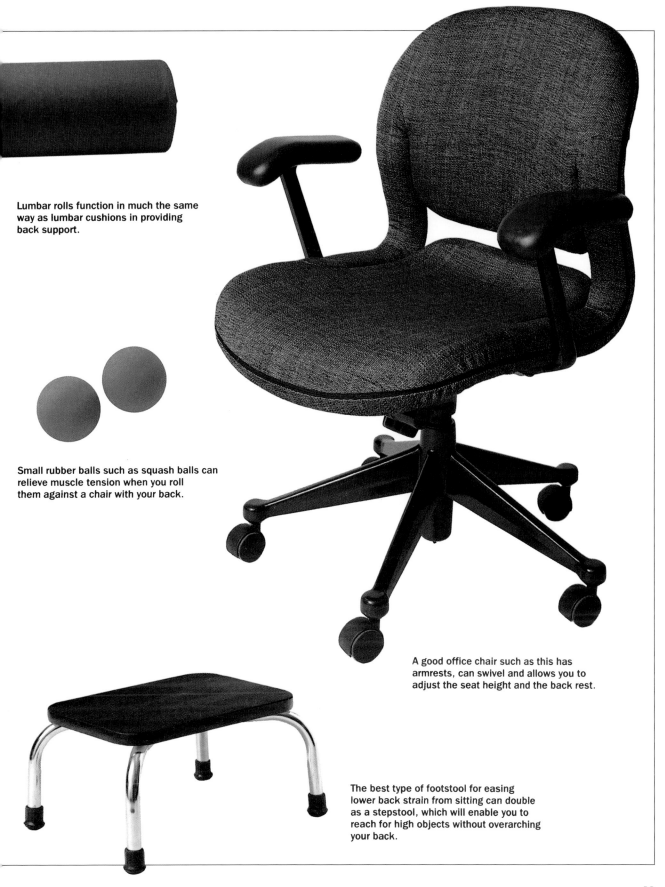

Lumbar rolls function in much the same way as lumbar cushions in providing back support.

Small rubber balls such as squash balls can relieve muscle tension when you roll them against a chair with your back.

A good office chair such as this has armrests, can swivel and allows you to adjust the seat height and the back rest.

The best type of footstool for easing lower back strain from sitting can double as a stepstool, which will enable you to reach for high objects without overarching your back.

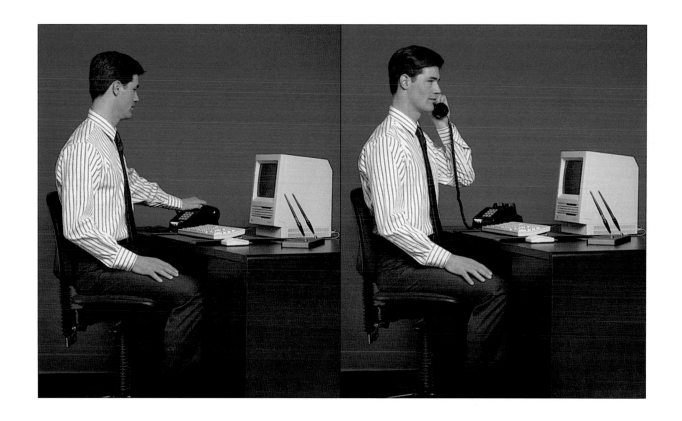

In the Office

Position your office phone on your left side if you are right-handed, and vice versa. It should be less than an arm's length away from your usual sitting position. As you reach for the receiver, keep your back resting against the chair and your torso aligned *(above)*. Bring the phone all the way up to your ear, keeping your head erect as you talk *(above, right)* or use a phone clip, as shown on the preceding page.

A dapting your office environment to accommodate your back can greatly reduce the stress of a sedentary job. Choosing the correct furniture, such as the chairs shown on the preceding two pages, is essential. It is crucial that whatever furniture you use should be adjusted to your body proportions. The curve in the back of your chair should conform to your lumbar curve, and the chair seat should be set so that your knees are at least as high as your hips when your feet rest on the floor. The height of your desktop should be slightly above your waist when you are seated.

Frequent telephone use can pose some problems, especially if you are writing or reaching for something while holding the receiver. The correct body mechanics, as shown above and on the right, help you avoid unnecessary twisting in such situations. In addition, you should endeavour to place the phone in an accessible spot so that you can reach anything that you may need while you are talking. The proper placement and use of other equipment, such as computers, typewriters and adding machines, can also ease potential back strain. If you are using a video display terminal, position it so that you need move only your eyes when you are looking from the keyboard to the terminal, allowing your head to remain still.

Take frequent breaks from sitting. Simply standing or taking a short walk will help release tension and avoid flexibility problems, as will performing the seated stretches that are shown on pages 66-67.

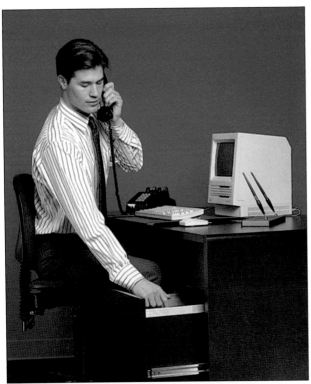

When reaching for something while you are on the phone, do not simply lean towards the object, but rotate your entire upper torso and bend forwards from the hips.

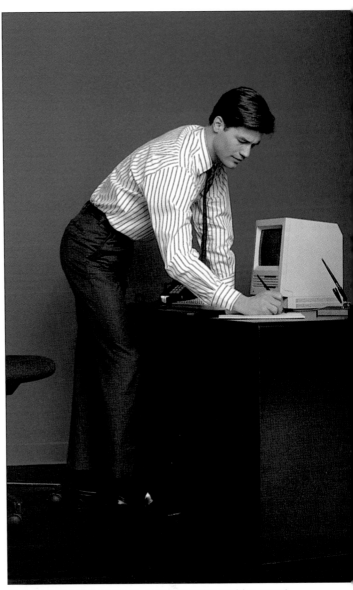

To lean over a desk and write from a standing position, stand with your feet shoulder-width apart in a lunge position. Rather than simply bending from the waist, lower your entire body by bending your knees and flexing at the hips.

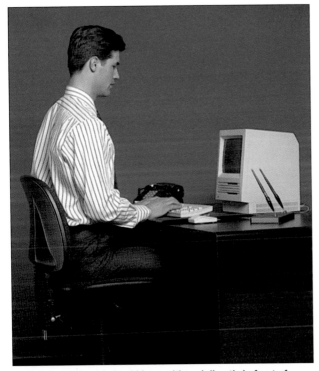

A desktop keyboard should be positioned directly in front of you. Rest your back against the chair and keep your arms at your sides, elbows slightly bent. Use your wrists and hands.

Daily Activity

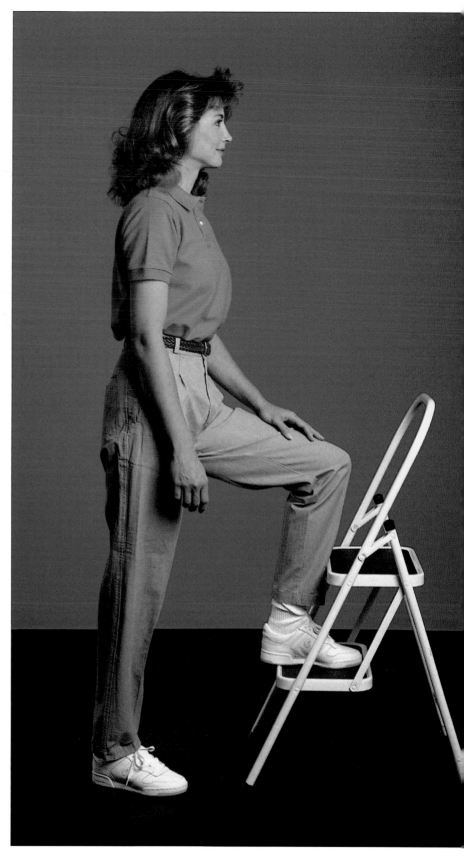

Using your back appropriately in everyday activities simply requires an awareness of how you move and, when necessary, making adjustments. For example, with many activities, haphazard movements can exaggerate the curve of the lower back, leading to back fatigue and possible injury. Such simple adjustments as bending your knees or using a stool can help to straighten the lower back, making it less prone to injury.

Virtually all of the activities you perform — from carrying a briefcase to doing housework to reading in bed — utilize six basic movements: sitting, standing, reclining, lifting, bending and reaching. Guidelines for these six are outlined here and on the following 12 pages; each basic movement is followed by several illustrated applications. This page, for example, demonstrates the correct technique for standing. The opposite page illustrates how to stand while cooking, putting on make-up or shaving, and brushing your teeth.

STANDING: When you stand for more than a few minutes, your vertebrae tend to sink down on themselves, which can make your lower back arch excessively. To avoid this, place one foot on a stool, book or any other similar object. Having one leg higher than the other will flatten the spinal curve.

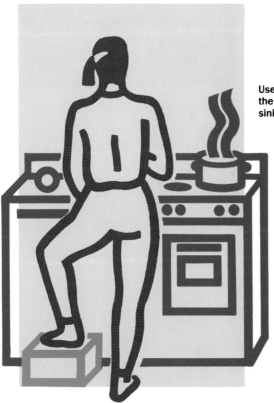

Use a stool or other footrest in the kitchen for the times you spend standing at the stove, sink or countertop.

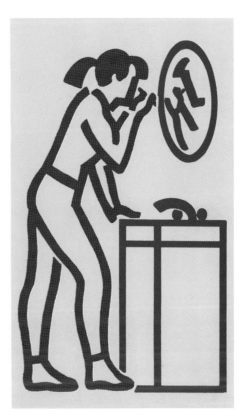

When leaning towards a mirror to apply make-up or to shave, stand in a lunging position and bend from the hips, keeping your back straight.

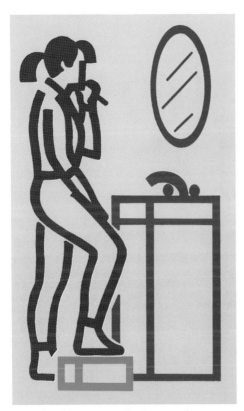

When brushing your teeth, place one foot on a stool. Bend forwards from the hips when leaning over the basin.

Lifting

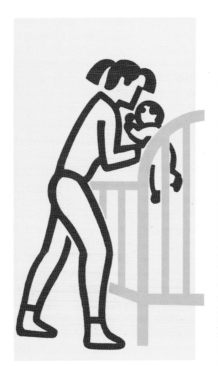

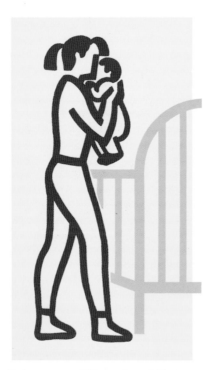

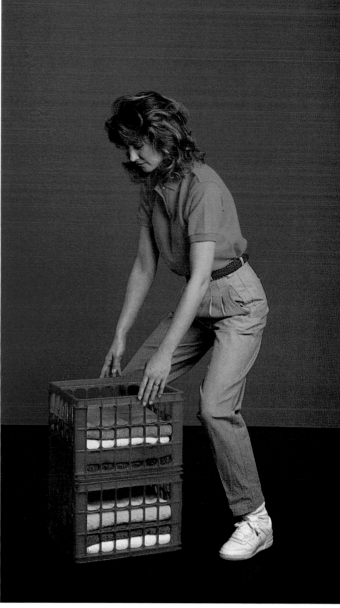

To lean over and lift, as when picking up a baby, assume a lunging position and bend from the hips *(top)*. Bring the baby close to you; then straighten up *(above)*.

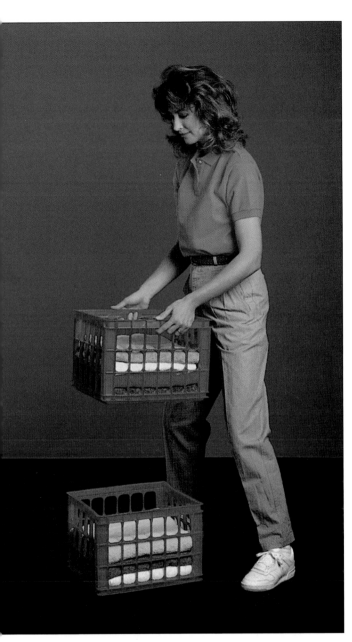

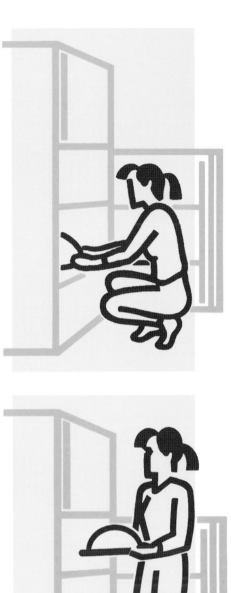

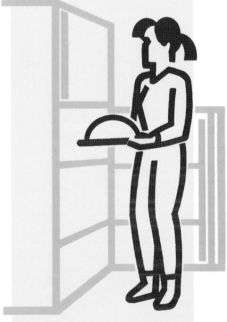

Proper positioning is an essential element of lifting. Stand close to the object you intend to lift and provide a broad base of support by spreading your feet wide on either side of it. Lower yourself by bending your knees, keeping your back aligned *(above, left)*. Hold the object close to you as you straighten your legs to return to a standing position *(above)*.

To lift and twist, squat *(top)* and pull the item towards you. Keep your knees and hips slightly bent as you turn and then rise *(above)*.

Carrying

Centring the load makes carrying easier. Keep your feet apart for a wide base and bend your knees slightly. Hold the object close to your torso so it can be supported by your body as well as your arms.

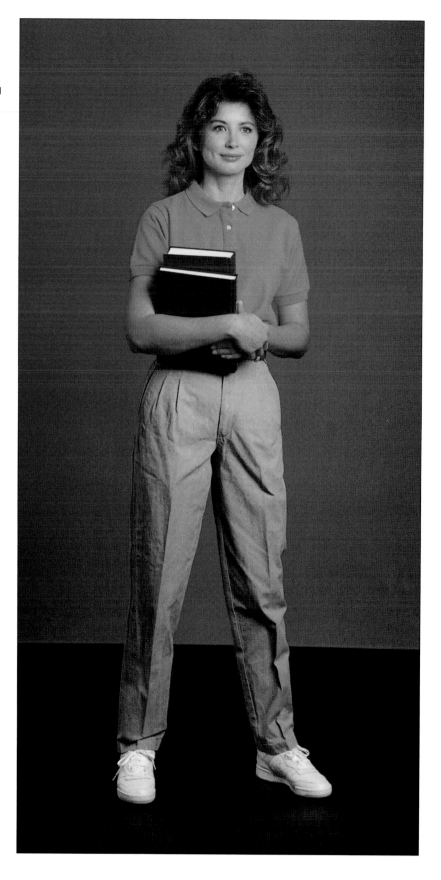

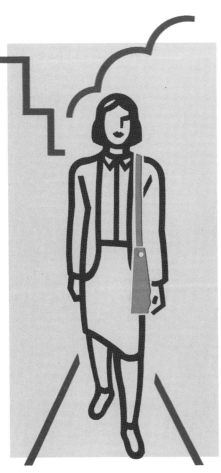

A briefcase with a shoulder strap helps spread the burden of weight to the upper torso. Adjust the strap length so that you can put a hand underneath the briefcase to provide additional support. Switch sides periodically to relieve the weight.

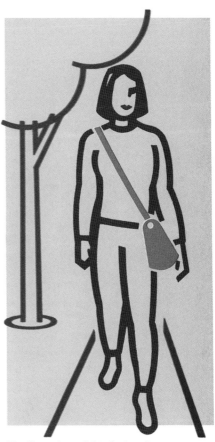

Distribute the weight of a handbag evenly on both sides of your body by carrying it with the strap across your chest. Place one hand underneath and hold it for extra support.

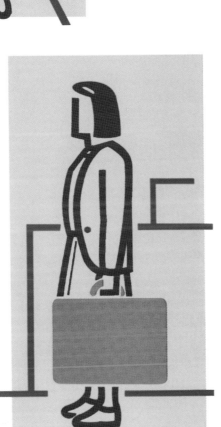

When you carry luggage, it is best to divide the weight evenly between two small suitcases. Otherwise, when carrying one large item, try to keep your shoulders level and provide a broad base with your feet. Alternate sides frequently.

Sitting

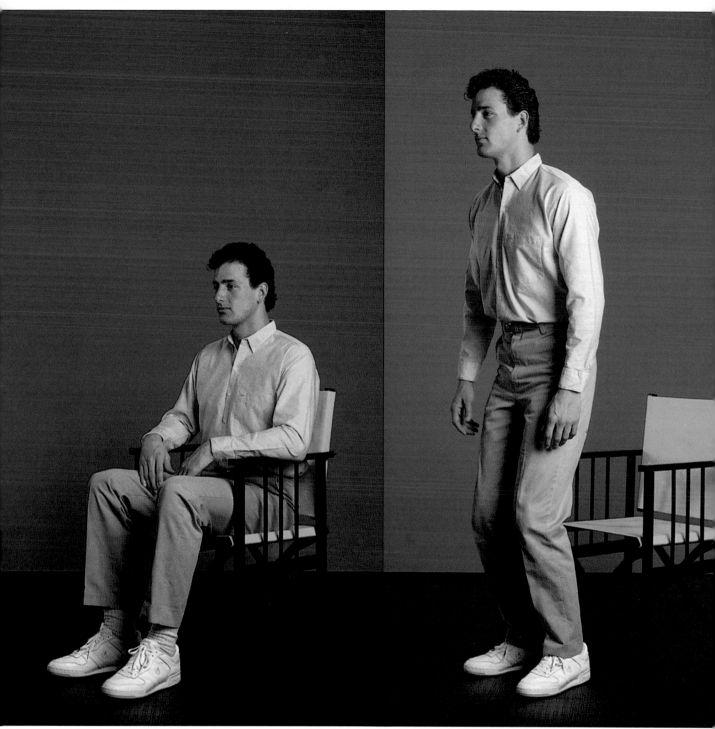

Sit all the way against the back of your chair. If the chair has
arms, lean your arms on them for support *(above)*. To stand
up, move to the edge of your chair and lean forwards from
your hips. Lead yourself out of the chair with your head,
keeping your entire torso aligned *(above, right)*.

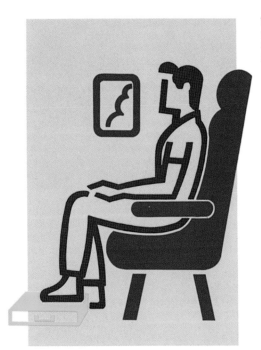

When travelling by plane or train, prop one foot on a piece of luggage. Alternate feet every 10 to 15 minutes to reduce lumbar compression.

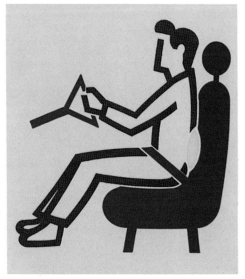

Position your car seat so that your elbows are bent when you hold the steering wheel and your knees are slightly bent when reaching the floor pedals. Support your lower back with a small pillow or lumbar cushion to keep your torso alignment almost vertical.

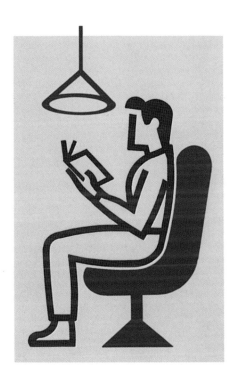

To read while seated, hold the book up at about chest level; avoid slumping forwards. If your arms grow tired, place a pillow on your lap to support the book.

Bending

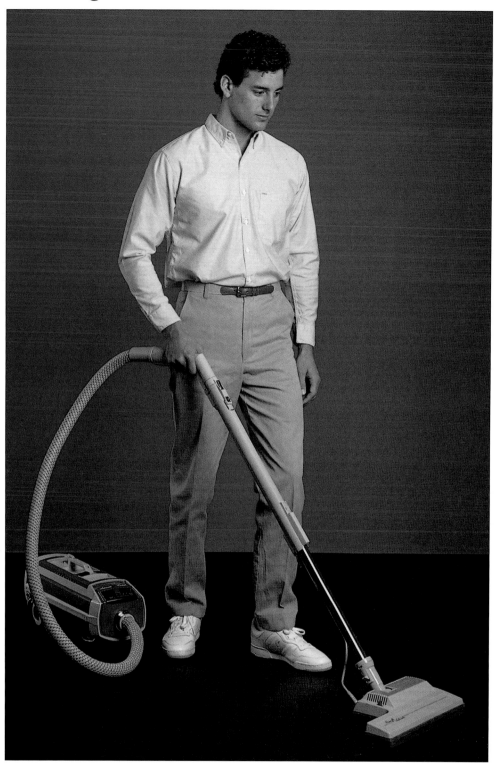

For housework and gardening that require bending and leaning, let your legs do the majority of the work. When vacuuming, for example, stand with your feet shoulder-width apart. Place one foot in front of the other and move back and forth by shifting your weight from foot to foot. Bend from the hips to lower your torso.

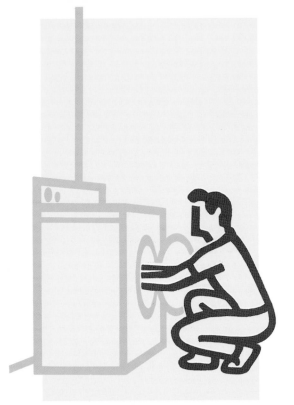

To reach into a dryer or dishwasher, lower your whole upper body by bending your knees and squatting.

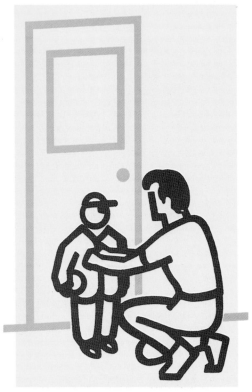

Use the same method as on the left to button a child's coat. You can rest one knee on the floor for more support.

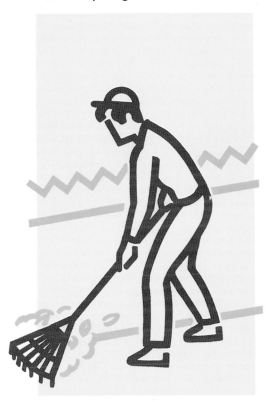

Use your feet as a broad base when raking. Reach down and forwards by flexing your hips, keeping your spine aligned.

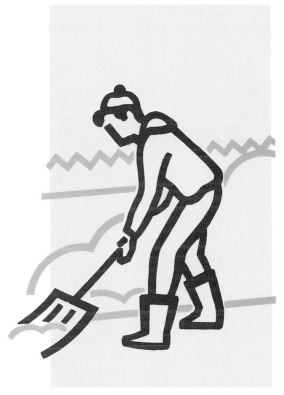

Place your hands well apart on a snow shovel to increase leverage. Bend at the hips to align your torso.

In Bed

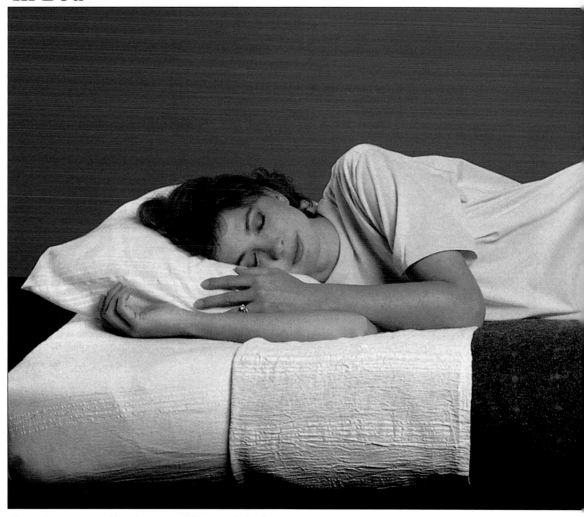

If you sleep on your side, place a semi-firm, good-sized pillow beneath your head and neck. Bend your knees and bring them up towards your chest. Place another pillow between your thighs and knees to reduce the pull exerted on your lower back by the upper legs.

Lying on your stomach is the worst position for your back, because it encourages arching of the lower back. If you must use this position, place a large pillow underneath your abdomen and bend one knee, bringing it up to the pillow. Do not use a pillow for your head.

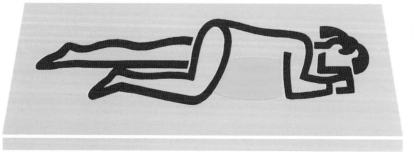

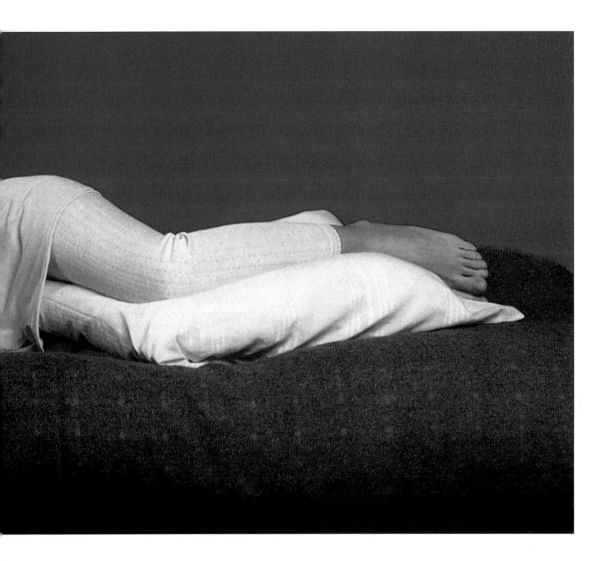

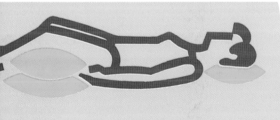

When sleeping on your back, place one or two good-sized pillows under your knees to reduce the curve in your lower back. Your head and neck should be supported by another pillow.

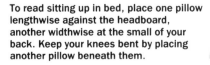

To read sitting up in bed, place one pillow lengthwise against the headboard, another widthwise at the small of your back. Keep your knees bent by placing another pillow beneath them.

Reaching

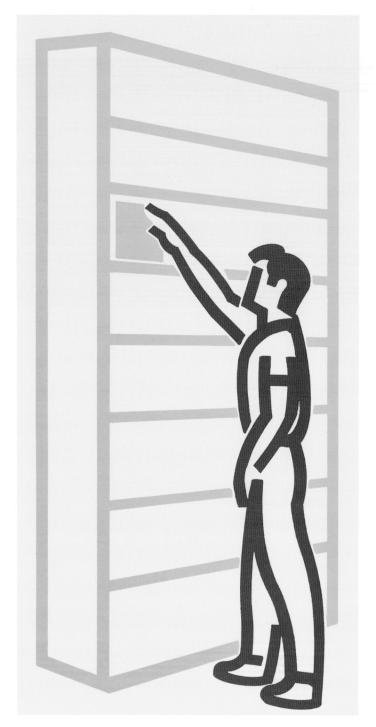

To reach for something placed above your head, stand within arm's length of the object in a lunge. The object should be low enough to reach without arching your lower back *(left)*. Otherwise, stand on a stool to avoid overextending your arm and back *(below)*.

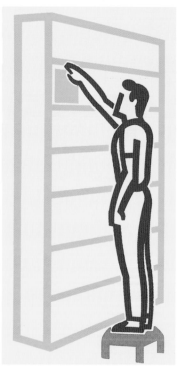

Socks and Shoes

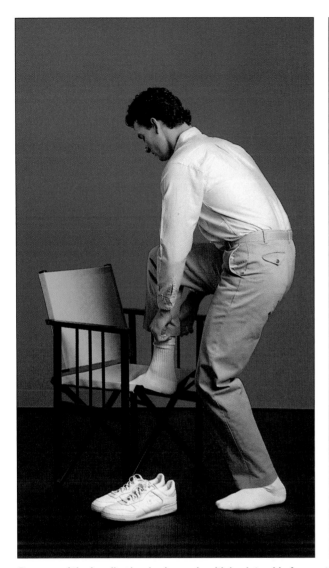 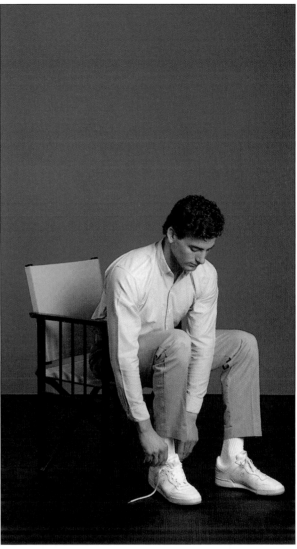

Because of the bending involved, people with back trouble frequently have problems getting dressed or undressed, particularly when reaching to their lower legs. To put on socks, raise one foot on to a chair or bed. Bend your other knee and lean forwards from your hips, keeping your spine and neck aligned *(above)*. Switch legs and repeat. Sit down and bend forwards from the hips to put your shoes on or take them off *(right)*.

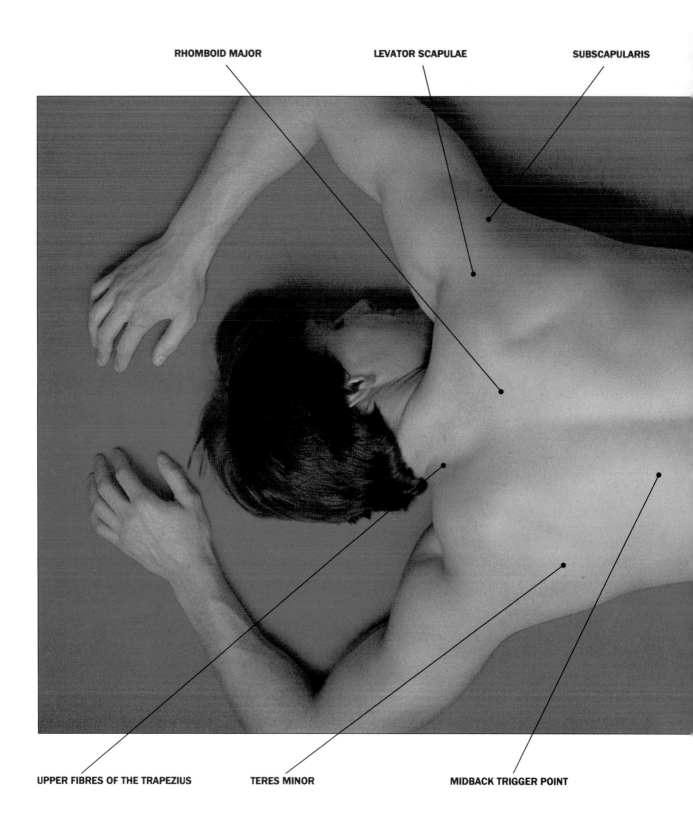

RHOMBOID MAJOR

LEVATOR SCAPULAE

SUBSCAPULARIS

UPPER FIBRES OF THE TRAPEZIUS

TERES MINOR

MIDBACK TRIGGER POINT

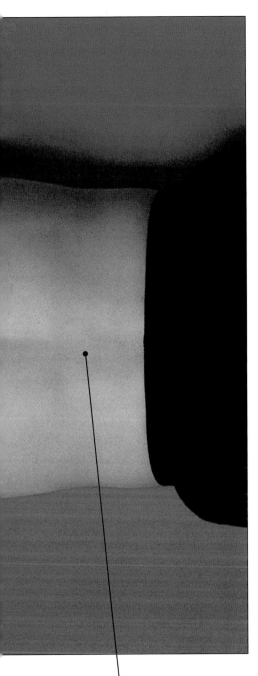

LOWER BACK TRIGGER POINT

Trigger Points

One way to alleviate back pain is to treat trigger points, which are specific locations deep within a muscle in which by-products of exertion not flushed out by the circulatory system can collect. Both stress and trauma can cause trigger points to become painful. In addition, poor posture as well as repetitive movements that lead to chronic muscle pain can irritate trigger points.

With the help of a friend, you can treat your trigger points both to prevent back-muscle tension and to relieve existing pain. Use the guide on the left to find which trigger points correspond to potentially troublesome muscles. Because of localized muscle tension and spasm, many trigger points feel like small nodules, which will help guide you and your partner to them.

Pressure on trigger points may feel uncomfortable but should not produce acute pain. In fact, you should feel relief immediately after a trigger point treatment. If a trigger point is especially sensitive, ask your partner to exert less pressure on it. Coordinating your partner's pressure with your breathing can also help to lessen the pain: your partner should exert pressure when you exhale and lighten pressure when you inhale. Repeated treatments of gradually increasing pressure may be needed for certain trigger points.

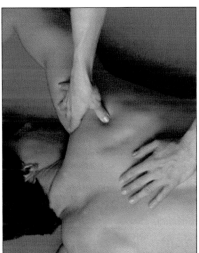

Kneel next to your partner. Use the ball of your thumb to apply pressure to a trigger point. Lean over so that you can use the weight of your upper body for added pressure. Spread your fingers to form a base and place your other hand nearby for support. Maintain the pressure for 10 to 15 seconds.

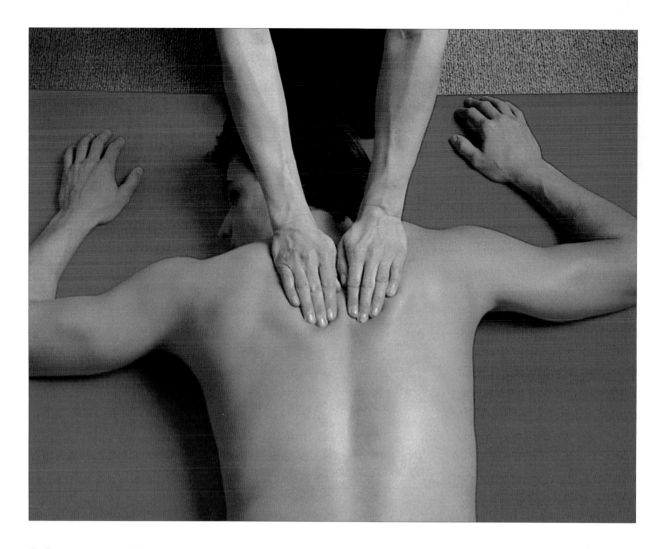

Massage/1

The relaxation that massage induces is more than merely superficial. Because a good massage can have such important physiological benefits, massage therapy has gained increased acceptance in recent years as part of muscle rehabilitation programmes for some back pain victims.

Massage dilates blood vessels, thereby stimulating circulation. The result is a cleansing process in which waste materials that have collected in the muscles and created pain are flushed out. If you are suffering from acute pain, only a licensed professional should attempt massage. However, if you are not in pain, you can attain some of the benefits of massage by asking a partner to perform on you the sequence shown here and on pages 120-123.

To prepare for a massage, lie on a mat in a warm room. Your partner should work deeply into your muscles, but never to the point of causing any pain; also, massage should never put any pressure directly on the spine. As the massage progresses, your skin will redden. Called hyperaemia, this painless condition is due to the increase in circulation and is indicative of the overall effectiveness of the massage.

Kneel at your partner's head and place your hands flat on either side of the spine. Stroke firmly straight down the back to the hip bones. Lightly glide your hands back to the neck, keeping your fingertips on the back. Repeat five times.

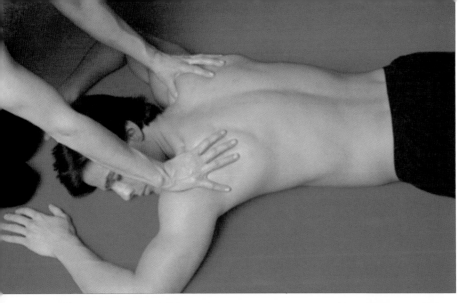

Place your thumbs on either side of the base of your partner's neck and spread your fingers as a base. Stroke outwards and back along the top of the shoulders, pressing deeply into the muscle. Repeat five times.

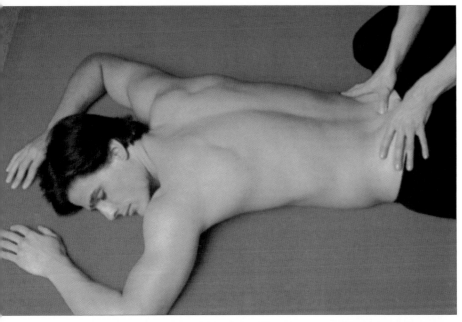

Straddle your partner's legs and place your thumbs on the sacrum, at the base of the spine. Spread your fingers. Rotate your thumbs in small circles, moving around to cover the entire sacrum.

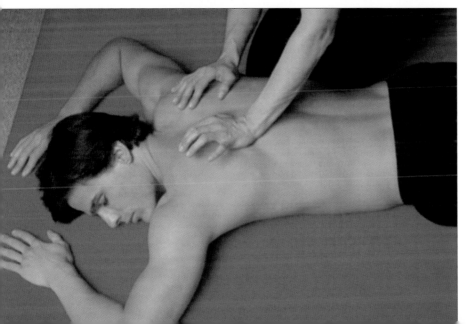

Move to your partner's side. Place one hand on the far side of the spine; rest your other hand on the upper back for support. Starting at the base of the neck, rotate your palm in small circles and push the muscle away from the spine. Work to the top of the buttocks. Perform two repetitions. Then switch arms and work on the side of the back closest to you, this time pulling towards you and away from the spine.

119

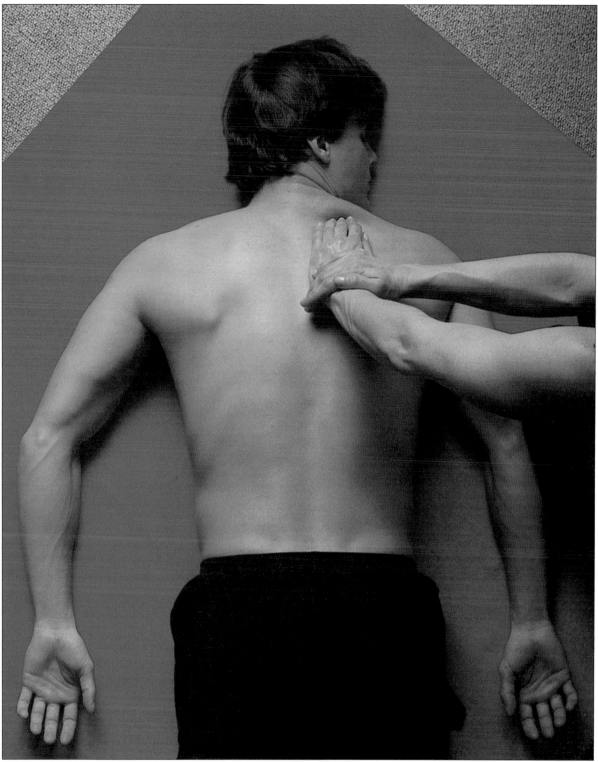

Massage/2

Place one hand on top of the other and make broad circles round the shoulder blade, pressing with your palm. Do not press on the bone itself or on the spine. Repeat five times. Switch shoulders and repeat.

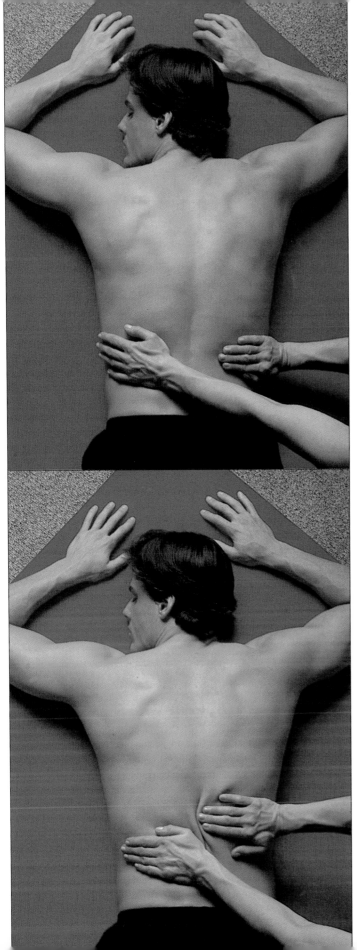

Place your hands on either side of your partner's waist *(left)*. Pressing with your palms, bring your hands towards each other *(below)*, avoiding pressure as they cross the spine. Your hands should end in the opposite position from where they started. Repeat this alternating, crossing motion as you work upwards to the shoulders, then back down again. Perform two repetitions.

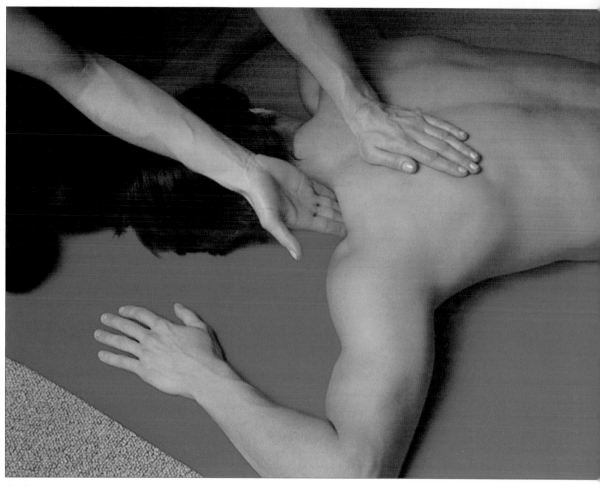

Massage/3

Move back to your partner's head. Put
your left hand on his left shoulder for
support. Place the fingertips of your right
hand beneath your partner's left shoulder.
Stroke along the inside of the shoulder
(above), up the neck to the base of the
skull, twisting your wrist as you work up
the neck *(above, right)*. Return and repeat
five times, then work up the other side.

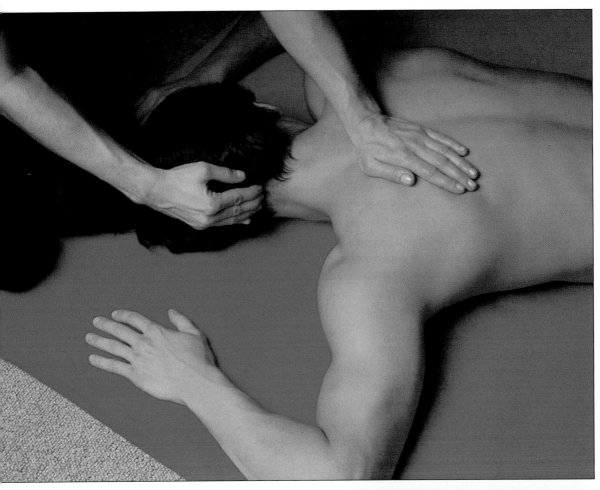

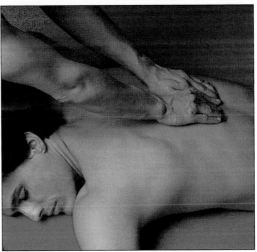

Finish the massage by repeating the first stroke, shown on page 118, down either side of the spine.

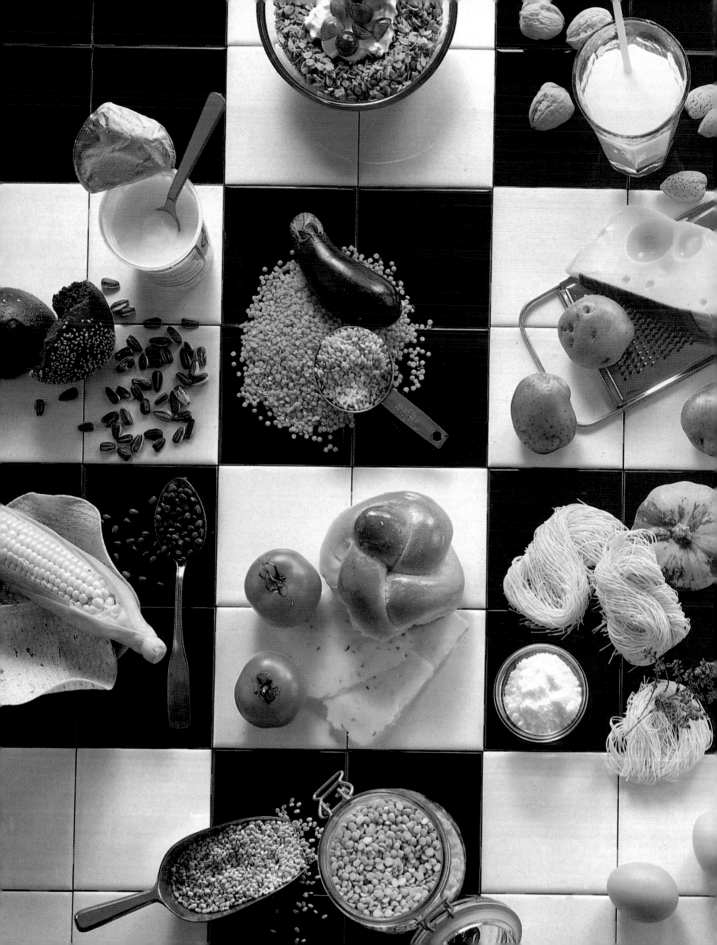

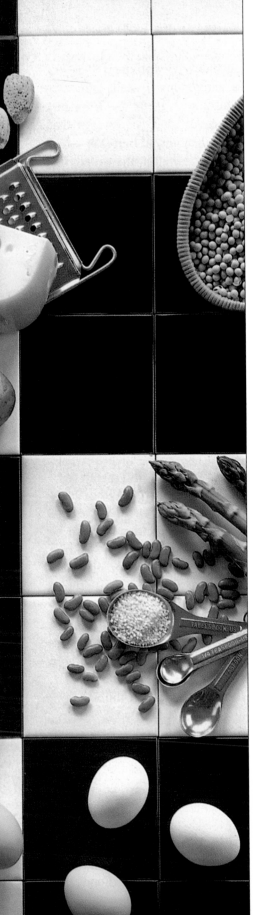

CHAPTER FIVE

Diet and Your Back

The right way to eat to minimize back problems

Although being overweight does not automatically condemn you to an aching back, extra weight can put added stress on your back in several ways. Carrying excessive body fat can result in bad posture, which may make the lower back particularly vulnerable to pain or injury. Studies show that because overweight people exercise less often than people of average weight, their middle-body muscles tend to be less flexible and more flaccid, which tends to put extra stress on the spine. Controlling your weight with both diet and exercise is therefore one of the best strategies you can adopt for avoiding back problems.

The key to an effective weight-control diet is restricting your intake of fat. And because red meat is a major source of fat in the diet of many people, substituting low-fat meatless recipes for some or all of the meat dishes you usually consume can help you lose weight, maintain a desired weight and reduce your risk of developing cardiovascular disease. Dishes devoid of red meat, poultry and fish are

125

generally lower in fat — weight for weight — than any other type of dish, and thus lower in calories.

A modified vegetarian regime that includes dairy products and eggs, as well as fruits, vegetables, pulses and grains, is called an ovo-lactovegetarian diet. Such a diet remains low in fat as long as its dairy products are based on skimmed or semi-skimmed milk, rather than whole milk, and it limits vegetable shortening, oil and butter — which together contribute up to 40 per cent of dietary fat in the British diet — as well as nuts. One recent study in the United States comparing 92 ovo-lactovegetarians and 113 meat eaters showed that the vegetarians weighed 7 kilograms less than the meat eaters, on average, when such factors as height and body structure were taken into account. Part of this weight advantage may be also be due to a difference in lifestyle, since people who choose to be ovo-lactovegetarians tend to be more active and more diet-conscious than most meat eaters.

In addition to reducing calorie intake, cutting out red meat can lower serum cholesterol levels. A survey of 116 men and women indicated that the vegetarians had blood cholesterol levels that averaged 33 per cent lower than the non-vegetarians. To maintain a level of blood cholesterol that minimizes your risk of heart attacks and strokes, you should restrict your consumption of egg yolks as well as red meat. One egg yolk contains approximately 300 milligrams of cholesterol, the amount recommended by the World Health Organization as the daily maximum for an adult.

Ovo-lactovegetarians eating a varied and balanced diet do not need to worry about nutritional deficiencies of calcium and vitamin B_{12}, which are sometimes lacking in the diet of pure vegetarians or vegans. However, getting enough iron on an ovo-lactovegetarian diet can be a problem. Eating vegetables such as spinach, chard and beetroot greens, which contain iron, can help. If you cut back or eliminate meat from your diet, you will find that some of the best low-fat protein substitutes are pulses, which include the mature or dried seeds of pod-bearing plants, such as lentils, split peas and kidney beans. Like most other plant-derived foods, pulses contain unsaturated fat, which is associated with reducing elevated blood cholesterol levels. Saturated fats, found chiefly in animal products such as meat, eggs and milk fat, are associated with high blood pressure, diabetes and the elevated cholesterol levels that are implicated in heart disease.

Pulses by themselves are abundant sources of many vitamins and minerals, but with the exception of soya beans, they are not complete proteins since they lack one of the nine essential amino acids, the basic units of protein that cannot be synthesized by the body and must be obtained from food. Combining pulses with any grain or seed or a small amount of animal protein can provide the complete protein that the body needs to build and maintain muscles, organs and antibodies. For example, in the Lentil Taboulleh in Pitta Pockets on page 132, combining lentils with burghul provides complete protein. Foods that

The Basic Guidelines

For a moderately active adult, Britain's National Advisory Committee on Nutrition Education recommends a diet that is low in fat, high in carbohydrates and moderate in protein. The committee's proposals for the long term suggest that no more than 30 per cent of your calories come from fat, that around 11 per cent come from protein and hence that 55 to 60 per cent come from carbohydrates. A gram of fat equals nine calories, while a gram of protein or carbohydrate equals four calories; therefore, if you eat 2,100 calories a day, you should consume approximately 70 grams of fat, 310 grams of carbohydrate and 60 grams of protein daily. If you follow a low-fat/high-carbohydrate diet, your chance of developing heart disease, cancer and other life-threatening diseases may be considerably reduced.

◆ The nutrition charts that accompany each of the low-fat/high-carbohydrate recipes in this book include the number of calories per serving, the number of grams of fat, carbohydrate and protein in a serving, and the percentage of calories derived from each of these nutrients. In addition, the charts provide the amount of calcium, iron and sodium per serving.

◆ Calcium deficiency may be associated with periodontal diseases — which attack the mouth's bones and tissues, including the gums — in both men and women, and with osteoporosis, or bone shrinking and weakening, in elderly women. The deficiency may also contribute to high blood pressure. The daily allowance for calcium recommended by the United Kingdom Department of Health and Social Security (DHSS) is 500 milligrams a day for men and women. Pregnant and lactating women are advised to consume 1,200 milligrams daily.

◆ Although one way you can reduce your fat intake is to cut your consumption of red meat, you should make sure that you get your necessary iron from other sources. The DHSS suggests a minimum of 10 milligrams of iron per day for men and 12 milligrams for women between the ages of 18 and 54.

◆ High sodium intake is associated with high blood pressure in susceptible people. Most adults should restrict sodium intake to about 2,000 milligrams a day, according to the World Health Organization. One way to keep sodium consumption in check is not to add table salt to food.

combine to provide all of the essential amino acids are called complementary proteins. The Peach Muffins on page 130, in which grains from the cereal and flour are complemented by the eggs and milk, and the Blue Cheese Spread with Tortilla Triangles on page 141, in which corn tortillas combine with cheese, provide complete protein.

The ovo-lactovegetarian dishes included in this chapter can form the basis of a low-calorie eating programme that may help you to control or lower your weight and thereby help safeguard your back. Carbohydrates and protein contribute more than 80 per cent of the calories in the recipes, while fat accounts for less than 25 per cent. Besides being low in fat and mostly cholesterol-free, such dishes also confer several other nutritional advantages. They are high in fibre, the edible but indigestible part of plants that aids in digestion and other bodily functions and that may contribute to weight control; and they contain all the important vitamins and minerals.

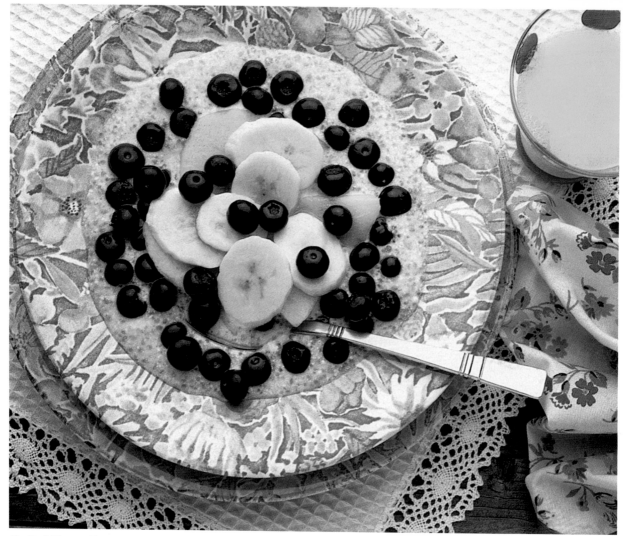

Fruited Ricotta Tapioca

Breakfast

FRUITED RICOTTA TAPIOCA

A pleasant change from cereal, this fruit-topped breakfast pudding is a good low-fat source of calcium, potassium and vitamins A and C.

CALORIES per serving	285
70% Carbohydrate	51 g
13% Protein	10 g
17% Fat	6 g
CALCIUM	191 mg
IRON	1 mg
SODIUM	116 mg

15 cl (¼ pint) apple juice concentrate
4 tablespoons quick-cooking tapioca
250 g (8 oz) low-fat ricotta cheese
2 large egg whites

1 tablespoon brown sugar
1 mango
1 banana
150 g (5 oz) fresh or frozen blueberries

Mix the apple juice, tapioca and 25 cl (8 fl oz) of water in a small pan and set aside for 5 minutes. Bring the mixture to the boil, stirring occasionally, and cook for 1 minute; remove the pan from the heat and set aside for 30 minutes, or until cool to the touch. Meanwhile, in a medium-sized bowl, whisk together the ricotta, egg whites and sugar until smooth. Fold the ricotta mixture into the tapioca and spoon the mixture into four dessert bowls. Cover the bowls with plastic film and refrigerate overnight.

Just before serving, stone the mango and cut it into 1 cm (½ inch) thick slices. Peel the banana and cut it into 5 mm (¼ inch) thick slices. Garnish the tapioca with the mango, banana and blueberries. *Makes 4 servings*

RASPBERRY-RICE SHAKE

This meal-in-a-glass gives you about the same amount of protein as two rashers of bacon and two eggs, but it has only about one fifth the fat. This shake also supplies 10 grams of fibre, while bacon and eggs have none.

CALORIES per serving	455
78% Carbohydrate	92 g
13% Protein	16 g
9% Fat	5 g
CALCIUM	433 mg
IRON	2 mg
SODIUM	153 mg

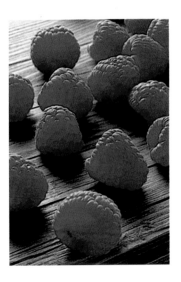

75 g (2½ oz) cooked brown rice
(30 g/1 oz raw weight)
1 banana, peeled
125 g (4 oz) frozen raspberries

17.5 cl (6 fl oz) plain low-fat yogurt
4 tablespoons skimmed milk
2 teaspoons honey

Place the rice in a food processor or blender and process until puréed, scraping down the sides of the container with a rubber spatula as necessary. Add the banana and process for another 30 seconds, or until the mixture is as smooth as possible. Add the raspberries, yogurt, milk and honey, and process for 15 seconds, or until blended. Serve immediately. *Makes 1 serving*

APPLE-RICE PANCAKE

Many people eat high-fat fast-food breakfasts for the sake of convenience, but this dense, crusty rice cake, which will keep for up to three days in the refrigerator, is just as convenient and much lower in fat.

300 g (10 oz) cooked white rice
(125 g/4 oz raw weight)
2 large eggs plus 1 egg white
2 tablespoons honey
1 Granny Smith apple

¼ teaspoon ground cinnamon
¼ teaspoon pure vanilla extract
¼ teaspoon grated lemon rind
2 teaspoons vegetable oil

In a medium-sized bowl, stir together the rice, eggs plus egg white and honey; set aside. Wash and core but do not peel the apple, then grate it into a small bowl and squeeze it dry. Add the apple, cinnamon, vanilla extract and lemon rind to the rice mixture and stir to combine.

Heat 1 teaspoon of the oil in a medium-sized frying pan over medium heat. Add the rice mixture and pat it into an even layer. Cover the pan and cook the mixture for 5 minutes, or until the bottom of the pancake is golden and the top is dry. To turn over the pancake, slide it on to a plate, cover with another plate and invert. Heat the remaining oil in the pan. Slide in the pancake cooked side up and reduce the heat. Cook the pancake, uncovered, for about 5 minutes, or until golden and cooked through. Cut into quarters and serve warm, or cool the pancake, refrigerate it and serve cold. *Makes 4 servings*

CALORIES per serving	230
69% Carbohydrate	39 g
10% Protein	6 g
21% Fat	5 g
CALCIUM	30 mg
IRON	2 mg
SODIUM	48 mg

PEACH MUFFINS

CALORIES per muffin	140
70% Carbohydrate	26 g
10% Protein	4 g
20% Fat	3 g
CALCIUM	50 mg
IRON	2 mg
SODIUM	153 mg

Although made with little fat, these muffins are so moist they can be eaten without butter or jam, which could add 50 to 100 calories.

30 g (1 oz) bran cereal
175 g (6 oz) plain flour
60 g (2 oz) wholemeal flour
1 teaspoon baking powder
1 teaspoon bicarbonate of soda
¼ teaspoon ground cinnamon

35 cl (12 fl oz) buttermilk
3 tablespoons vegetable oil
4 tablespoons honey
2 large eggs, lightly beaten
275 g (9 oz) dried peaches,
   coarsely diced

Preheat the oven to 190°C (375°F or Mark 5). Line an 18-hole bun tin with paper liners. In a large bowl, stir together the cereal, the flours, baking powder, bicarbonate of soda and cinnamon, and make a well in the centre. In a medium-sized bowl, beat together the buttermilk, oil, honey and eggs. Pour the buttermilk mixture into the dry ingredients, add the peaches and stir just to combine. Divide the batter among the bun tin cups and bake for 20 to 25 minutes, or until the muffins are lightly browned.   Makes 18 muffins

BLUEBERRY-ORANGE MILK SHAKE

CALORIES per serving	105
77% Carbohydrate	21 g
18% Protein	5 g
5% Fat	1 g
CALCIUM	190 mg
IRON	Trace
SODIUM	64 mg

Skimmed milk and fruit make this recipe an excellent low-fat source of the minerals calcium and potassium.

1 navel orange
100 g (3 ½ oz) frozen blueberries

25 cl (8 fl oz) skimmed milk

Grate 2 teaspoons of rind from the orange, being careful not to include any of the white pith; set aside. Peel and segment the orange; remove and discard the membranes. Place the segments in a polythene bag and freeze them for 3 to 4 hours, or until frozen solid.

Place the blueberries, the orange segments and rind in a food processor or blender and process until puréed, scraping down the sides of the container with a rubber spatula. Add the milk and process for 1 minute, or until well blended. Pour the shake into two tall glasses and serve.   Makes 2 servings

QUICK BROWN RICE PUDDING

CALORIES per serving	205
82% Carbohydrate	42 g
11% Protein	6 g
7% Fat	2 g
CALCIUM	158 mg
IRON	2 mg
SODIUM	46 mg

Instead of cereal and milk, try this breakfast "pudding". It is a better source of protein and fibre than most packaged cereals. You can cook rice especially for this recipe, or use leftover rice.

12.5 cl (4 fl oz) plain low-fat
   yogurt
1½ teaspoons molasses
1 teaspoon honey

½ teaspoon pure vanilla extract
150 g (5 oz) cooked brown rice
   (60 g/2 oz raw weight)
2 tablespoons currants

In a small bowl, mix the yogurt, molasses, honey and vanilla extract. Stir in the rice and currants. Chill before serving, if desired.   Makes 2 servings

Lunch

HERBED POTATOES AU GRATIN

Potatoes baked with cheese can be loaded with fat, but this version gets its flavour from herbs and onions, and uses just 2 tablespoons of cheese.

750 g (1½ lb) new potatoes
15 g (½ oz) butter
1 tablespoon plain flour
4 tablespoons chopped parsley
1½ teaspoons fresh rosemary
1 teaspoon crushed garlic

¼ teaspoon black pepper
35 cl (12 fl oz) skimmed milk
90 g (3 oz) onion, sliced
2 tablespoons grated
   Emmenthal cheese

CALORIES per serving	225
69% Carbohydrate	39 g
14% Protein	8 g
17% Fat	4 g
CALCIUM	171 mg
IRON	2 mg
SODIUM	130 mg

Preheat the oven to 190°C (375°F or Mark 5). Slice the unpeeled potatoes 5 mm (¼ inch) thick and place them in a bowl of cold water. Melt the butter in a small saucepan over medium-low heat. Stir in the flour, half the parsley, the rosemary, garlic and black pepper. Gradually add the milk, stirring until thick and smooth; set the sauce aside.

Drain and dry the potatoes; put half in a 22 cm (9 inch) round casserole and top with half the onion. Repeat the layers with the remaining potatoes and onion. Pour on the sauce, cover the dish with foil and bake for 30 minutes. Stir gently and bake for 30 minutes more. Stir again, sprinkle on the cheese and bake, uncovered, for 10 to 15 minutes, or until the cheese is golden-brown. Sprinkle with the remaining parsley and serve.   Makes 4 servings

Herbed Potatoes au Gratin

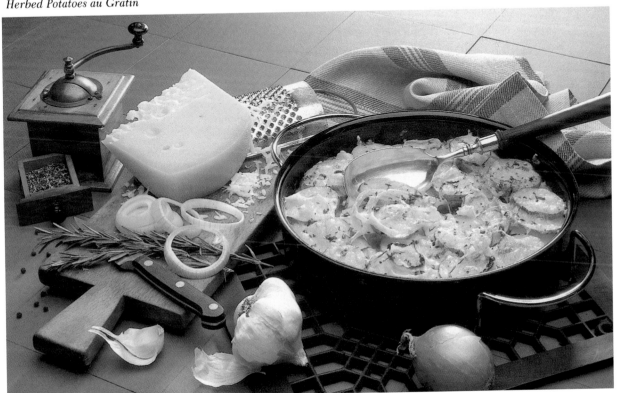

VEGETABLE-BRIE MELT

Creamy-tasting Brie gives this sandwich a rich taste, but the topping consists mainly of vegetables, with less than 15 g (½ oz) of cheese per serving.

CALORIES per serving	210
65% Carbohydrate	34 g
15% Protein	8 g
20% Fat	5 g
CALCIUM	80 mg
IRON	3 mg
SODIUM	506 mg

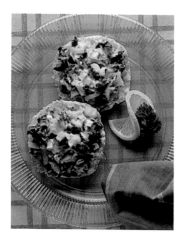

90 g (3 oz) spinach, shredded
125 g (4 oz) carrots, grated
45 g (1½ oz) mushrooms, coarsely chopped
60 g (2 oz) shallots, coarsely chopped

45 g (1½ oz) Brie cheese, chilled and finely diced
4 tablespoons plain low-fat yogurt
1 tablespoon Dijon mustard
¼ teaspoon black pepper
4 muffins

Preheat the oven to 190°C (375°F or Mark 5). In a medium-sized bowl, mix the spinach, carrots, mushrooms, shallots, Brie, yogurt, mustard and pepper, and stir with a wooden spoon until well blended; set aside. Split and toast the muffins, and place them cut side up on a baking sheet. Spoon some of the vegetable mixture on each muffin half and bake for 10 minutes, or until heated through. Divide among four plates and serve.　　　Makes 4 servings

LENTIL TABOULLEH IN PITTA POCKETS

The combination of lentils, a pulse, and burghul, a whole grain, makes these sandwiches an excellent low-fat source of protein and iron.

200 g (7 oz) lentils
175 g (6 oz) onion, diced
2 garlic cloves, crushed
125 g (4 oz) burghul
60 g (2 oz) parsley, finely chopped
60 g (2 oz) fresh mint, finely chopped
1½ teaspoons dried thyme
1½ teaspoons dried oregano

Tabasco sauce
1 tablespoon vegetable oil
1 teaspoon grated lemon rind
Eight 30 g (1 oz) pitta breads
1 small cucumber
60 g (2 oz) feta cheese, rinsed and drained
8 large cos lettuce leaves, torn into bite-sized pieces

CALORIES per serving	280
71% Carbohydrate	50 g
16% Protein	12 g
13% Fat	4 g
CALCIUM	103 mg
IRON	5 mg
SODIUM	276 mg

Place the lentils, onion, garlic and 75 cl (1¼ pints) of water in a medium-sized saucepan and cook over medium heat for 30 minutes, or until the lentils are tender. Stir in the burghul, then add half the parsley and mint, and cook over low heat for 2 minutes. Add the thyme, oregano, and Tabasco sauce to taste, then cover the saucepan, remove it from the heat and set it aside to cool to room temperature. (If the pan is not kept covered, the burghul will not absorb the liquid properly.)

When the lentil mixture is cool, pour off any excess liquid from the pan, pressing the mixture gently with a slotted spoon. (It should be firm enough to retain the impression of the spoon.) Transfer the mixture to a bowl and stir in the remaining mint and parsley, the oil and lemon rind. Cover the bowl and refrigerate the mixture for at least 2 hours, or until well chilled.

Just before serving, wrap the pitta breads in foil and warm them in a low oven. Meanwhile, peel, seed and thinly slice the cucumber and finely dice the feta cheese. Cut open one end of each pitta bread. Place some lettuce in each pitta. Divide the lentil mixture equally among the pockets and top with some of the feta and cucumber.　　　Makes 8 servings

CREAM OF TOMATO SOUP WITH CROUTONS

This soup has the same amount of protein as canned tomato soup prepared with whole milk, but one sixth the fat and half the sodium.

CALORIES per serving	125
78% Carbohydrate	26 g
16% Protein	5 g
6% Fat	1 g
CALCIUM	112 mg
IRON	2 mg
SODIUM	441 mg

400 g (14 oz) canned plum
   tomatoes, with their liquid
25 cl (8 fl oz) tomato juice
250 g (8 oz) new potatoes, peeled
   and diced
200 g (7 oz) sweet red peppers,
   diced

175 g (6 oz) onions, chopped
3 tablespoons chopped fresh
   coriander
1 garlic clove, crushed
¼ teaspoon pepper
1 slice wholemeal bread
17.5 cl (6 fl oz) skimmed milk

Preheat the oven to 190°C (375°F or Mark 5). In a medium-sized pan, mix the tomatoes and their liquid, the tomato juice, potatoes, red peppers, onions, 2 tablespoons of the coriander, the garlic and pepper, and bring to the boil. Cover the pan, reduce the heat to low and simmer for 15 minutes. Meanwhile, cut the bread into 1 cm (½ inch) cubes, spread them on a baking sheet and bake for 5 to 10 minutes, or until golden; set aside to cool.

Remove the soup from the heat and set aside to cool for a few minutes. Purée the soup in a food processor or blender for 1 minute, or until smooth. With the machine running, gradually add the milk. Return the soup to the pan and reheat over medium-high heat. Ladle the soup into four bowls, top it with the croutons and garnish with the remaining coriander.   Makes 4 servings

ASPARAGUS FRITTATA

Plenty of vegetables, very little oil and less than one egg per serving make this Italian-style omelette a filling and nutritious lunch.

CALORIES per serving	320
63% Carbohydrate	51 g
18% Protein	15 g
19% Fat	7 g
CALCIUM	120 mg
IRON	4 mg
SODIUM	522 mg

2 teaspoons olive oil
100 g (3½ oz) leeks, thinly sliced
300 g (10 oz) sweet red peppers,
   diced
90 g (3 oz) red onion, chopped
2 garlic cloves, crushed
500 g (1 lb) asparagus, cut into
   2.5 cm (1 inch) pieces, blanched
75 g (2½ oz) mushrooms, sliced
250 g (8 oz) unpeeled new
   potatoes, boiled and sliced

4 fresh plum tomatoes, peeled,
   seeded and chopped
4 large eggs
12.5 cl (4 fl oz) semi-skimmed
   milk
2 tablespoons grated Parmesan
4 tablespoons chopped parsley
½ teaspoon dried tarragon
½ teaspoon salt
¼ teaspoon pepper
350 g (12 oz) loaf Italian bread

Heat the oil in a large frying pan over medium heat. Sauté the leeks, peppers, onion and garlic for 5 minutes. Add the asparagus and mushrooms, and cook for 4 minutes. Then add the potatoes and tomatoes, and cook, stirring occasionally, for 3 minutes. Whisk the eggs, milk, Parmesan, herbs, salt and pepper in a bowl. Pour the mixture into the pan, lifting the vegetables so that the eggs flow underneath. Increase the heat to medium high and cook for 10 minutes, or until the eggs are almost set. Meanwhile, preheat the grill. Grill the frittata 15 cm (6 inches) from the heat for 1 minute, or until the top is lightly browned. Slice the bread. Carefully invert the frittata on to a platter, cut into six wedges and serve with the bread.   Makes 6 servings

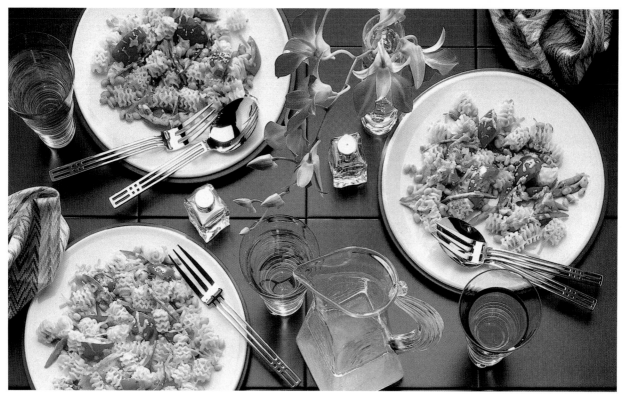

Soya Bean and Pasta Salad

Dinner

SOYA BEAN AND PASTA SALAD

Soya beans are among the best non-meat protein sources. Miso, a Japanese flavouring paste, is made from fermented soya beans.

CALORIES per serving	**325**
71% Carbohydrate	59 g
18% Protein	15 g
11% Fat	4 g
CALCIUM	107 mg
IRON	5 mg
SODIUM	155 mg

4 tablespoons dried soya beans,
  soaked overnight in cold water
500 g (1 lb) tomatoes
125 g (4 oz) carrots
125 g (4 oz) mange-tout
250 g (8 oz) pasta grills or spirals

4 teaspoons light miso
¼ teaspoon ground ginger
¼ teaspoon black pepper
4 tablespoons plain low-fat yogurt
1 tablespoon chopped parsley
1 teaspoon toasted sesame seeds

Drain the soya beans, add fresh cold water to cover them and bring them to the boil over medium heat. Cover the pan, reduce the heat to low and simmer for 1 hour, or until the beans are just tender. Skim off and discard the skins, which will float to the surface. While the beans are cooking, core the tomatoes and cut them into chunks. Trim, peel and grate the carrots. Trim the mange-tout. Bring a medium-sized saucepan of water to the boil and blanch the mange-tout for 30 seconds, or until they turn bright green; rinse them under cold running water and set them aside to drain.

Drain the soya beans and set them aside to cool. Bring a large pan of water to the boil. Cook the pasta for 10 minutes, or according to the packet directions, until *al dente*. Meanwhile, for the dressing, stir together the miso, ginger

134

and black pepper in a small bowl. Gradually stir in the yogurt, then add 4 tablespoons of cold water and stir until smoothly blended; set aside. Cut the mange-tout into slivers. When the pasta is done, drain it, rinse it under cold water and set it aside to drain thoroughly.

To serve, place the pasta, tomatoes, carrots, mange-tout and soya beans in a large bowl. Pour on the dressing, sprinkle the salad with the parsley and sesame seeds, and toss gently to combine.   Makes 4 servings

BEAN-STUFFED PARATHAS

These Indian griddle breads are low in fat because the dough contains less fat than usual. The spicy filling is very high in protein.

CALORIES per serving	425
69% Carbohydrate	76 g
16% Protein	17 g
15% Fat	7 g
CALCIUM	70 mg
IRON	5 mg
SODIUM	294 mg

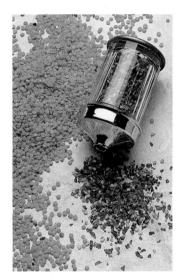

60 g (2 oz) dried chick-peas	1 tablespoon vinegar
100 g (3½ oz) red lentils	2 teaspoons honey
90 g (3 oz) onion, chopped	1 teaspoon ground cumin
1 low-sodium vegetable stock cube	⅓ teaspoon hot red pepper flakes
2 tablespoons finely chopped fresh ginger root	½ teaspoon salt
	125 g (4 oz) wholemeal flour
1½ tablespoons low-sodium tomato purée	150 g (5 oz) strong plain flour
	1½ tablespoons olive oil

Bring the chick-peas and 50 cl (16 fl oz) of water to a simmer in a medium-sized pan, and cook for 2 minutes. Cover the pan and refrigerate overnight.

Bring the chick-peas to the boil over medium heat, cover and cook for 15 minutes. Add the lentils, onion and stock cube, and simmer for 45 minutes. Reduce the heat to low, add the ginger, tomato purée, vinegar, honey, cumin, pepper and ¼ teaspoon salt, and cook, uncovered, stirring occasionally, for 10 minutes. Remove the pan from from the heat and set aside to cool.

For the dough, place the wholemeal flour, strong flour, 1 tablespoon of oil and the remaining salt in a food processor. With the machine running, add 15 cl (¼ pint) of water and process for 45 seconds, or until a smooth, elastic dough is formed. Place the dough in a polythene bag, close the top and set aside to rest in a warm place for about 30 minutes.

Lightly flour the work surface and roll out the dough into a 38 cm (15 inch) disc. Brush the dough with the remaining oil, then roll it into a log. With the rolling pin, flatten the log slightly, sealing the ends. Cut the log crosswise into 12 equal pieces. Place one piece of dough on the work surface and roll it out to a 12 cm (5 inch) disc. Place a scant 2 tablespoons of filling on the circle of dough, bring the edges together in the centre and pinch them to seal the paratha. Turn it over and flatten it to a 10 cm (4 inch) disc. Repeat with the remaining dough, placing the parathas on a sheet of greaseproof paper.

Heat a medium-sized frying pan over medium heat. Place three parathas at a time, seam side down, in the pan and cook for 5 minutes; turn and cook for 3 more minutes. Turn again and cook for another minute. Keep them warm while you cook the remaining parathas in the same fashion. Divide the parathas among four plates and serve.   Makes 4 servings

Note: you can make the parathas in advance and reheat them before serving. Place the parathas on a baking sheet, cover them with foil and heat in a 180°C (350°F or Mark 4) oven for 10 minutes.

PASTA WITH SWEET PEPPER-TOMATO SAUCE

CALORIES per serving	285
75% Carbohydrate	54 g
16% Protein	11 g
9% Fat	3 g
CALCIUM	153 mg
IRON	4 mg
SODIUM	292 mg

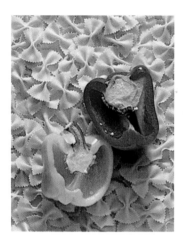

The nutritional benefits of pasta are enhanced by serving it with a low-fat sauce and a modest amount of cheese. With this method of making sauce — simmering all the ingredients together from the start — neither oil nor butter is needed to sauté the onion and garlic.

400 g (14 oz) canned plum tomatoes, with their liquid	¼ teaspoon coarsely ground black pepper
175 g (6 oz) onions, coarsely chopped	Pinch of salt
3 garlic cloves, crushed	2 large sweet yellow or red peppers, slivered
4 tablespoons chopped fresh basil	250 g (8 oz) farfalle (bow-tie) pasta
1 bay leaf	4 tablespoons grated Parmesan

For the sauce, mix the tomatoes and their liquid, the onions, garlic, basil, bay leaf, black pepper and salt in a medium-sized pan, and bring to the boil over medium heat, breaking up the tomatoes with a wooden spoon. Reduce the heat to medium low and simmer the sauce, uncovered, for 15 minutes.

Add the sweet peppers, cover the pan and simmer for 15 minutes more. Meanwhile, bring a large pan of water to the boil. Cook the pasta for 10 minutes, or according to the packet directions, until *al dente*. Drain the pasta and divide it among four plates. Remove and discard the bay leaf from the sauce. Spoon the sauce over the pasta, then sprinkle 1 tablespoon of Parmesan over each portion and serve. Makes 4 servings

POLENTA WEDGES

CALORIES per serving	280
67% Carbohydrate	47 g
14% Protein	10 g
19% Fat	6 g
CALCIUM	272 mg
IRON	1 mg
SODIUM	255 mg

This version of polenta, an Italish dish made from cooked, cooled cornmeal, is low in fat and high in protein and supplies a good amount of calcium. Serve it with a salad for a satisfying dinner.

60 cl (1 pint) semi-skimmed milk	100 g (3 ½ oz) sultanas
90 g (3 oz) cornmeal	¼ teaspoon salt
2 teaspoons margarine	Black pepper
½ teaspoon chopped fresh rosemary	4 tablespoons grated Emmenthal cheese

Heat the milk in a medium-sized heavy-bottomed saucepan over medium heat just to the boiling point. Whisk in the cornmeal in a thin, even stream. Reduce the heat to low and simmer, stirring, for about 5 minutes, or until thick. Stir in the margarine, rosemary, sultanas, salt, and pepper to taste, and transfer the mixture to a 22 cm (9 inch) pie plate. Let the polenta cool slightly, then cover it loosely with plastic film and refrigerate until thoroughly chilled. (The polenta may be made up to three days in advance and refrigerated.)

To serve, preheat the oven to 180°C (350°F or Mark 4). Cut four sheets of foil and lightly oil them. Slice the polenta into quarters, place one piece on each sheet of foil and sprinkle it with the grated Emmenthal cheese. Bake for 15 to 20 minutes, or until the polenta is thoroughly heated through and the cheese is melted and golden. Makes 4 servings

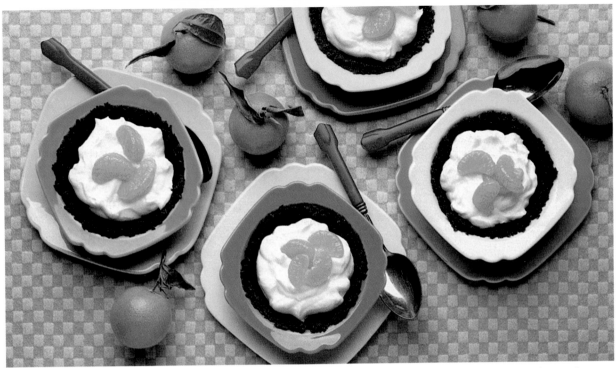

Cheesecake Cups

Dessert

CHEESECAKE CUPS

Cheesecake may derive 60 per cent of its calories from fat, with 15 grams per serving. One of these cheesecake cups has only 2 grams.

1 litre (1¾ pints) plain low-fat
   yogurt
3 tablespoons sugar
1 teaspoon grated lemon rind
1 teaspoon pure vanilla extract

2 slices pumpernickel bread
2 tablespoons honey
400 g (14 oz) canned juice-packed
   mandarin orange segments,
   drained

Line a large strainer with a triple thickness of damp muslin and place it over a medium-sized bowl. Gently spoon the yogurt into the strainer, cover it with plastic film and place in the refrigerator for 4 to 6 hours.

Leaving the yogurt in the strainer, stir in the sugar, lemon rind and vanilla extract, cover and refrigerate for another 4 to 6 hours, or overnight. You should have about 50 cl (16 fl oz) of yogurt cheese, depending on the type of yogurt used and the length of time it is drained.

Preheat the oven to 190°C (375°F or Mark 5). For the crust, toast the bread in the oven for 10 to 15 minutes, or until dry. Process the bread in a food processor or blender until it is reduced to crumbs. Add the honey and process for another 5 seconds, or until blended. Divide the mixture among eight dessert bowls or ramekins and press it into the base of each one to form a crust. Spoon a scant 4 tablespoons of the yogurt cheese into each cup. Decorate with the orange segments and serve.

Makes 8 servings

CALORIES per serving	140
69% Carbohydrate	24 g
19% Protein	7 g
12% Fat	2 g
CALCIUM	218 mg
IRON	4 mg
SODIUM	127 mg

PEACH YOGURT FREEZE

CALORIES per serving	180
75% Carbohydrate	34 g
16% Protein	7 g
9% Fat	2 g
CALCIUM	222 mg
IRON	1 mg
SODIUM	89 mg

Although commercial frozen yogurts are usually low in fat, they may be loaded with sugar. When you make your own, you can control the sugar content, relying on the natural flavour of fruit for sweetness.

500 g (1 lb) canned water-packed peaches, drained
25 cl (8 fl oz) plain low-fat yogurt
1 teaspoon pure vanilla extract

1 tablespoon brown sugar
2 dried apricot halves, cut into thin strips

Place the peaches, yogurt, vanilla and sugar in a food processor or blender and process for 1 minute, or until smooth. Spoon the mixture into two dessert bowls and cover with plastic film. Freeze the mixture, stirring occasionally to break up the ice crystals, for 2 hours, or until frozen but still soft. Just before serving, garnish each portion with the apricots.   Makes 2 servings

APPLE STRUDEL

CALORIES per serving	340
77% Carbohydrate	67 g
6% Protein	5 g
17% Fat	7 g
CALCIUM	32 mg
IRON	2 mg
SODIUM	114 mg

While fatty foods produce a sensation of fullness, dietary fibre does the same thing with far fewer calories. Apples and prunes are rich sources of fibre.

150 g (5 oz) plain flour
4 tablespoons sugar
30 g (1 oz) margarine, well chilled
2 tart apples (about 300 g/10 oz)
¼ teaspoon lemon juice

10 stoned prunes, chopped
4 tablespoons dry breadcrumbs
¼ teaspoon ground cinnamon
⅛ teaspoon ground ginger

In a medium-sized bowl, stir together the flour and half of the sugar. Cut the margarine into small pieces, then using a pastry blender or two knives, cut the margarine into the dry ingredients until the mixture is crumbly. Stir in 2 to 3 tablespoons of iced water and mix to form a soft dough. Form the dough into a ball, wrap it in plastic film and refrigerate it for at least 30 minutes.

Meanwhile, wash, core and halve but do not peel the apples. Rub one apple half with the lemon juice, then wrap and refrigerate it for the garnish. Dice the remaining apples and place them in a medium-sized bowl. Add the chopped prunes, breadcrumbs, 1 tablespoon of sugar, ⅛ teaspoon of cinnamon and the ginger, and stir until well blended. Stir together the remaining sugar and cinnamon in a small bowl; set aside.

Preheat the oven to 180°C (350°F or Mark 4). Line a baking sheet with foil. Lightly dust the work surface and a rolling pin with flour, then roll out the dough to a 30 by 18 cm (12 by 7 inch) rectangle, dusting the surface with additional flour as necessary. Place the filling in the centre of the dough to form a 22 by 7.5 cm (9 by 3 inch) rectangle. Bring the long sides of the dough together, fold them over once and pinch them together to seal firmly. Fold in the ends and press firmly to seal them so that the filling does not leak out. Place the strudel seam side down on the baking sheet, sprinkle it with the cinnamon-sugar and bake for 25 minutes, or until it is lightly browned at the edges. Let the strudel cool on the baking sheet for 5 minutes. Meanwhile, cut the reserved apple half into eight slices. Cut the strudel into four pieces, garnish with the apple slices and serve.   Makes 4 servings

WHOLEMEAL PANCAKES WITH MIXED FRUIT

These fruit-filled pancakes need no heavy sauce or cream to top them, and a serving gives you more than your daily requirement of vitamin C.

125 g (4 oz) wholemeal flour

3 tablespoons sugar

3 large eggs

150 g (5 oz) frozen unsweetened blueberries, thawed and drained

2 oranges, peeled, halved and cut crosswise into thin slices

2 tablespoons honey

2 tablespoons lemon juice

¼ teaspoon ground cardamom

2 kiwi fruit, peeled, halved and thinly sliced

1 tablespoon vegetable oil

CALORIES per pancake	170
67% Carbohydrate	30 g
11% Protein	5 g
22% Fat	4 g
CALCIUM	40 mg
IRON	1 mg
SODIUM	29 mg

For the batter, process the flour, sugar, eggs and 35 cl (12 fl oz) of water in a food processor or blender for 1 minute. Transfer to a bowl, cover and refrigerate until needed. (The batter may be made up to 3 hours in advance.)

For the filling, mix the blueberries, orange slices, honey, lemon juice and cardamom in a medium-sized pan and cook over medium heat for 5 minutes, or until the fruit is slightly softened; transfer to a bowl. Drain the kiwi slices, add them to the bowl and toss gently; set aside at room temperature.

Preheat the oven to its lowest setting. To make the pancakes, stir the batter well to reblend it. Heat a medium-sized non-stick frying pan over medium-high heat and brush it lightly with oil. Pour in 4 tablespoons of the batter and swirl the pan to coat the bottom evenly. Cook the pancake for 1½ minutes, then turn it and cook for another 30 seconds. Transfer the cooked pancake to an ovenproof plate, cover it loosely with foil and place it in the oven to keep warm. Repeat to make a total of eight pancakes.

Lay each pancake browned side down on a dessert plate, spoon on about 4 tablespoons of the filling and fold the sides of the pancake over it. Top each pancake with a spoonful of the remaining filling.   Makes 8 servings

Note: the pancakes can be made in advance and frozen. To freeze, interleave them with sheets of greaseproof paper and wrap the stack tightly in foil. To thaw, remove the foil and paper, put the pancakes in a baking tin, cover with foil and warm in a 150°C (300°F or Mark 2) oven for about 10 minutes.

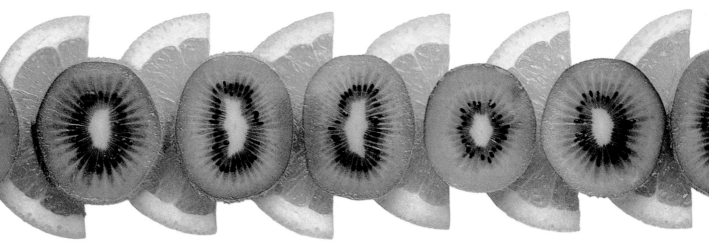

Snacks

STUFFED EGGS

A generous spoonful of spicy potato filling takes the place of the yolks in this version of devilled eggs. The yolks contain all the fat and cholesterol in eggs; almost all the protein is in the whites.

CALORIES per serving	100
72% Carbohydrate	18 g
20% Protein	5 g
8% Fat	1 g
CALCIUM	20 mg
IRON	1 mg
SODIUM	152 mg

500 g (1 lb) new potatoes
8 large eggs
1 small apple, peeled and cored
1 large stick celery
3 tablespoons chutney
2 tablespoons soured cream
2 tablespoons dry breadcrumbs

1 tablespoon chopped fresh chives
1½ teaspoons curry powder
¼ teaspoon salt
Tabasco sauce
¼ teaspoon paprika

Put the potatoes and eggs in a medium-sized pan with cold water to cover. Bring to the boil and cook for 12 minutes. With a slotted spoon, remove the eggs and cool them under cold running water. Cook the potatoes for 15 minutes more, then drain and cool for 15 minutes. Meanwhile, shell the eggs, halve them lengthwise and discard the yolks; set aside the whites.

Peel and quarter the potatoes, place them in a medium-sized bowl and mash them until smooth. Finely chop the apple and celery in a food processor or by hand, then add them to the mashed potatoes. Add the chutney, soured cream, breadcrumbs, 2 teaspoons of the chives, the curry powder, salt, and Tabasco sauce to taste and stir until well blended. Spoon the mixture into the egg whites and place them on a plate; cover with plastic film and refrigerate for at least 2 hours. Just before serving, garnish the eggs with the remaining chives and sprinkle them with the paprika.   Makes 8 servings

Stuffed Eggs

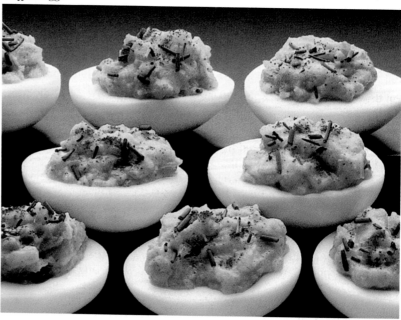

BROWN RICE BISCUITS

Commercial savoury biscuits, even "natural" whole-grain varieties, can derive 45 to 50 per cent of their calories from saturated fats.

2 tablespoons skimmed milk
1 tablespoon walnut oil
150 g (5 oz) cooked brown rice
   (60 g/2 oz raw weight)

125 g (4 oz) wholemeal flour
1 teaspoon salt
½ teaspoon coarsely ground
   black pepper

CALORIES per biscuit	25
70% Carbohydrate	5 g
11% Protein	1 g
19% Fat	1 g
CALCIUM	4 mg
IRON	Trace
SODIUM	74 mg

In a small bowl, stir together the milk, oil and 2 tablespoons of water; set aside. Place the rice, flour, salt and pepper in a food processor and process for 2 to 3 seconds, or just until mixed. With the machine running, add the milk mixture and process just until the dough forms a cohesive mass. If necessary, add up to 1 tablespoon more water. The dough will be sticky but should hold its shape when a small piece is pinched off. Form the dough into a ball, wrap it loosely in plastic film and set aside for 15 minutes.

Lightly flour the work surface and a rolling pin. Pat the dough into a disc, then roll it to a 1 cm (½ inch) thickness. Let it rest for 10 to 15 minutes, then roll it out again. Repeat the process twice, rolling the dough slightly thinner each time; dust with flour if necessary. Let the dough rest between rollings.

Preheat the oven to 180°C (350°F or Mark 4). Roll the dough out to a 25 by 22 cm (10 by 9 inch) rectangle about 3 mm (⅛ inch) thick. Using a ruler and a sharp knife, cut the dough into thirty 7.5 by 2.5 cm (3 by 1 inch) rectangles. Place the biscuits 1 cm (½ inch) apart on a baking sheet and bake for 20 minutes, or until crisp and golden. Transfer the biscuits to racks to cool and repeat with the remaining dough. *Makes 60 biscuits*

BLUE CHEESE SPREAD WITH TORTILLA TRIANGLES

The spread is potato-based and the tortillas are baked, making this a low-fat snack. And, because the complete protein in dairy products complements the incomplete protein in grains, you get more usable protein.

500 g (1 lb) new potatoes,
   scrubbed
Four 20 cm (8 inch) corn tortillas
12.5 cl (4 fl oz) skimmed milk
30 g (1 oz) blue cheese, crumbled

1 tablespoon chopped fresh
   chives
¼ teaspoon coarsely ground
   black pepper

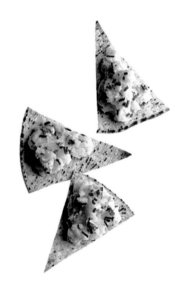

Put the potatoes in a medium-sized pan with cold water to cover and bring to the boil. Cover the pan, reduce the heat and simmer for 20 minutes, or until the potatoes are tender when pierced with a knife. Drain and set aside.

Meanwhile, preheat the oven to 240°C (475°F or Mark 9). Dip each tortilla in a bowl of water, then cut it into eight triangles. Place the triangles on a baking sheet and bake for 3 to 4 minutes, or until crisp. Remove the triangles from the oven and reduce the temperature to 150°C (300°F or Mark 2). Bake the triangles for 2 to 3 minutes more, or until golden-brown; set aside.

Peel and quarter the potatoes. Place them in a medium-sized bowl and mash them, then gradually stir in the milk, cheese, chives and pepper. The mixture should be well blended but not completely smooth. Transfer it to a serving bowl and serve with the tortilla triangles. *Makes 4 servings*

CALORIES per serving	195
71% Carbohydrate	35 g
14% Protein	7 g
15% Fat	3 g
CALCIUM	126 mg
IRON	2 mg
SODIUM	175 mg

ACKNOWLEDGEMENTS

The editors wish to thank Kate Cann and Norma MacMillan.

Nutritional analyses provided by Hill Nutrition Associates, New York State.

Index prepared by Ian Tucker.

Index

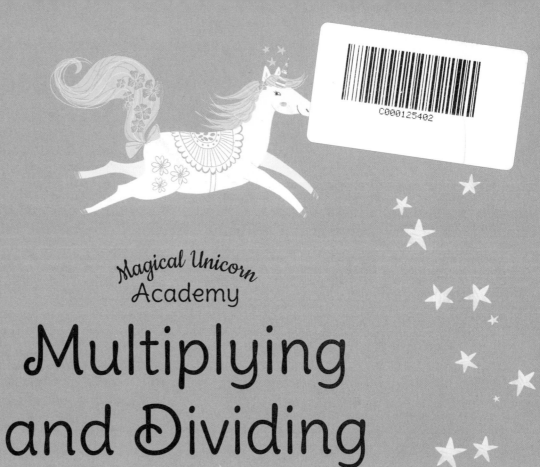

Magical Unicorn
Academy

Multiplying
and Dividing

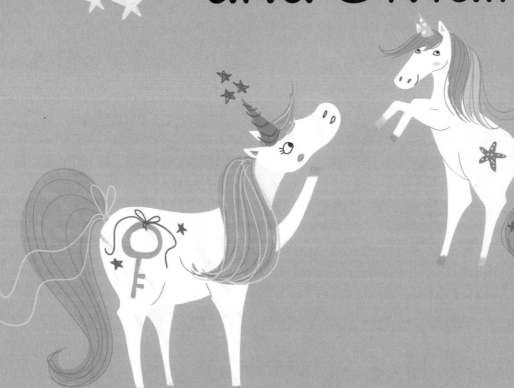

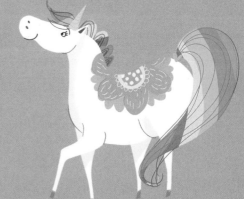

ARCTURUS

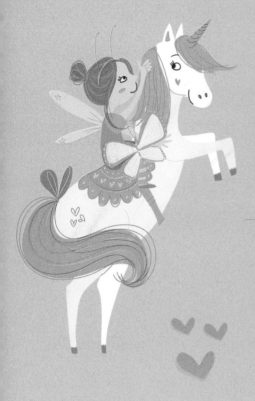

Key skills in this book

ARCTURUS

This edition published in 2022 by Arcturus Publishing Limited
26/27 Bickels Yard, 151–153 Bermondsey Street,
London SE1 3HA

Author: Lisa Regan
Illustrator: Sam Loman
Editors: Becca Clunes and Donna Gregory
Designer: Linda Storey
Managing Editor: Joe Harris

ISBN: 978-1-3988-0399-2
CH008632NT
Supplier 29, Date 1121, Print run 11798

Printed in China

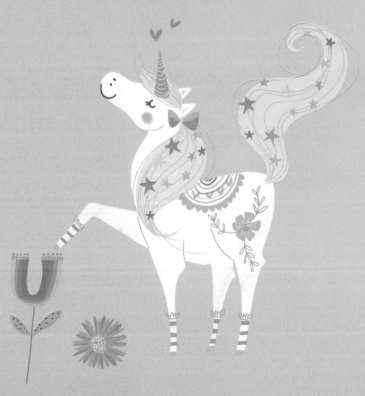

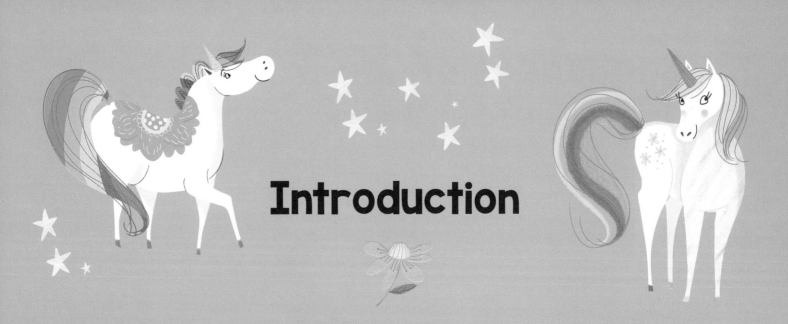

Introduction

Welcome to Magical Unicorn Academy! Join the unicorns and their enchanted friends as they set out to discover just how magical mathematics can be!

In this book, you'll find lots of fun activities that will help you multiply and divide any numbers. Start at the beginning, where you will learn all the times tables, and then work through the book. As you go, you'll discover all kinds of tips and tricks to help you get better and better at multiplication and division—even with big numbers! So grab your pencil, get your thinking cap on, and let's set off on a mathematics adventure!

Sequences of Ten

Fill in the missing numbers for each
unicorn by counting up in tens.

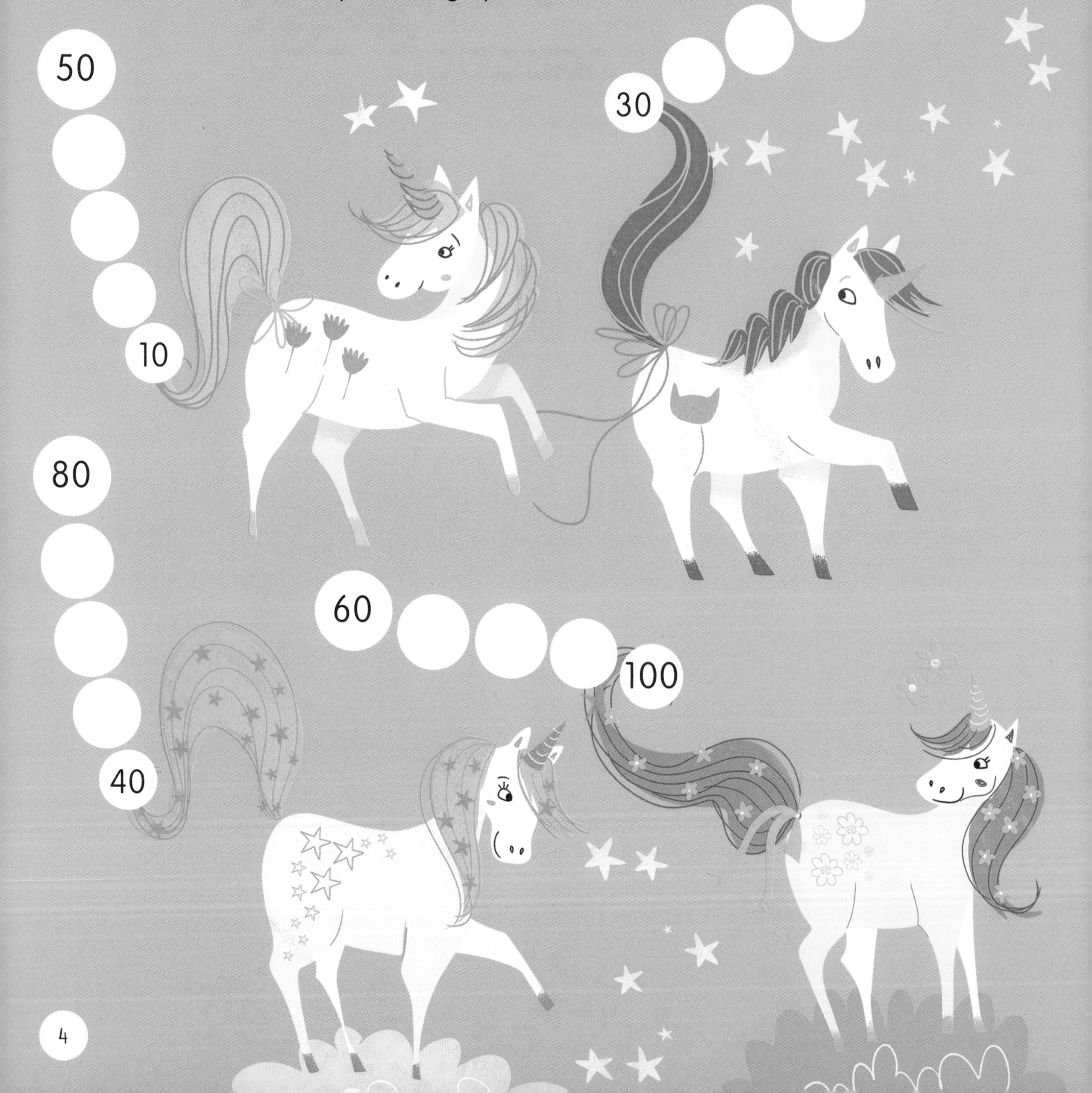

70

50

30

10

80

60

100

40

Sweet Treats

Count in fives to fill in the numbers
on all of these goodies.

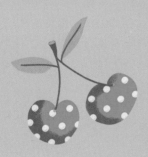 

 5  10   20   35

 20 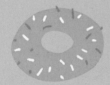  30 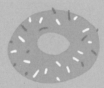 40 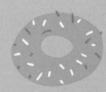 50

 40  35 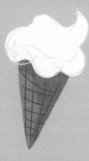 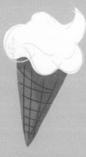 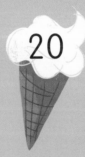 20 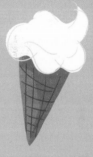 10

 80   90    110

Under the Sea

Find out who is swimming with
Missy Mermaid by joining the dots.
Count in twos to join them in the correct order.

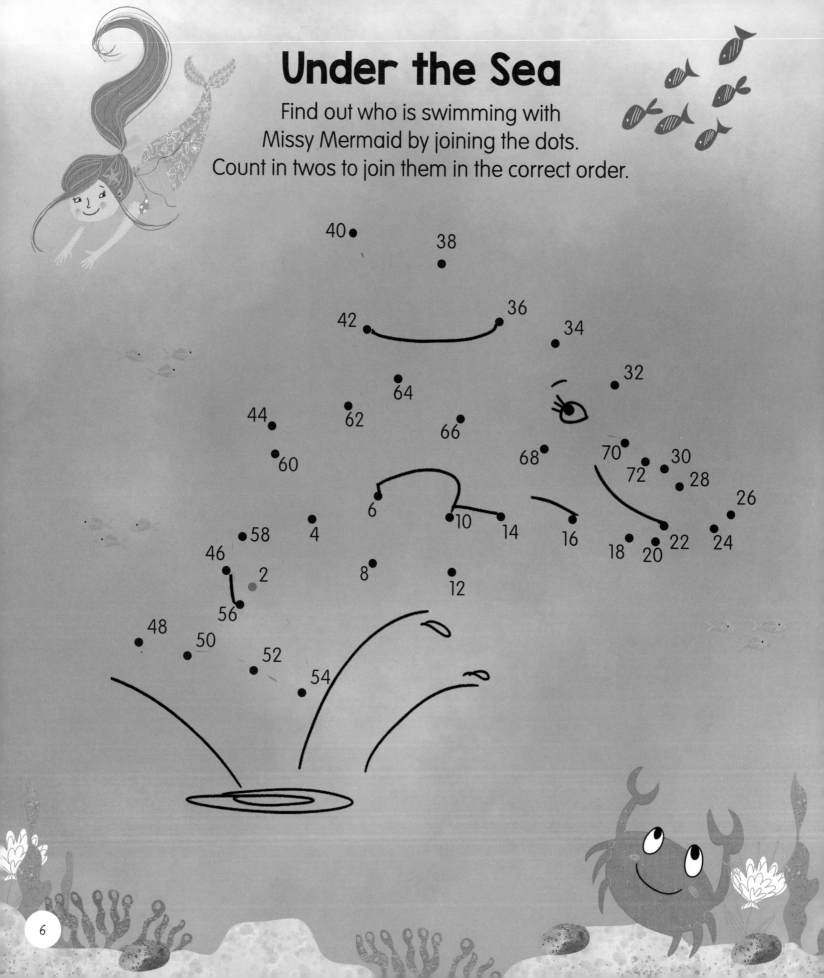

Totally Tropical

Work out the sequences and fill in the missing numbers each time.

2	4	6	8	10	
50	45	40	35	30	
100	90	80	70	60	
76	78	80	82	84	
45	50	55	60	65	

Again and Again

Use repeated addition to find out the number of creatures in each group. The first one shows you how to do it.

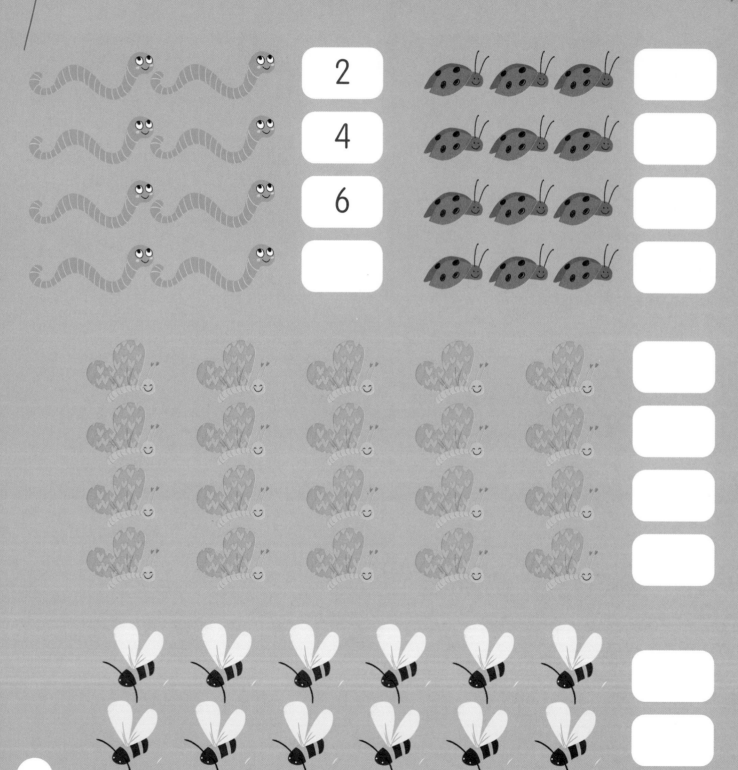

Now Multiply

This time, count the creatures using multiplication.
Count each column and row, then multiply them together.

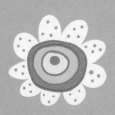
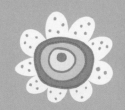
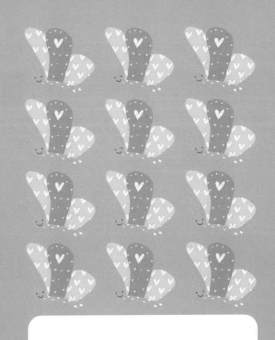

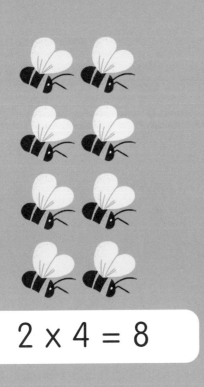

$$2 \times 4 = 8$$

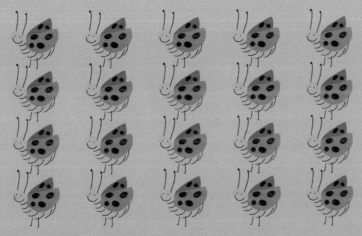

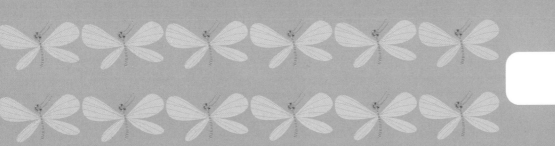

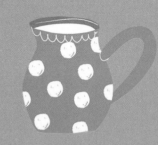

Food for Thought

Write the correct numbers in the blank space,
and then work out the answer. The first has
been done to show you how.

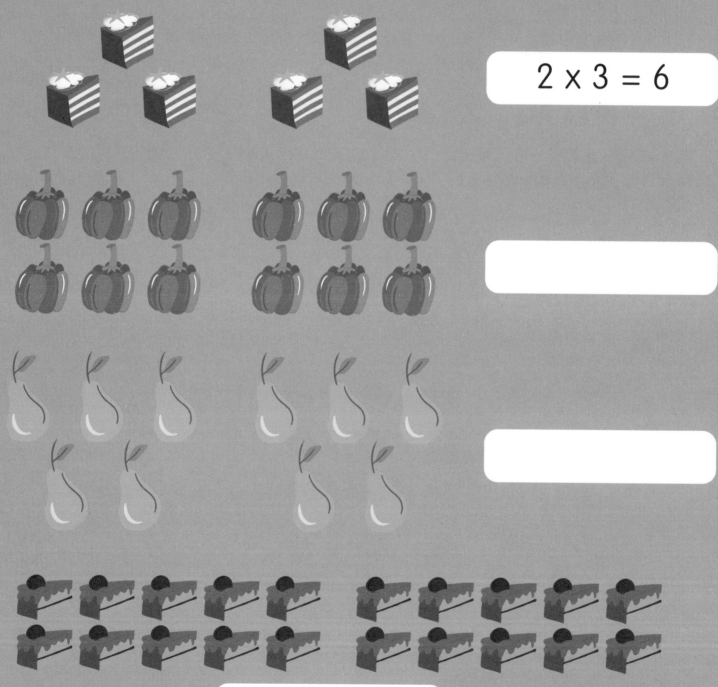

$2 \times 3 = 6$

More Food for Thought

Here are some more goodies for you to try!

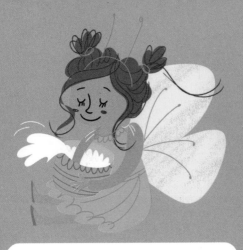

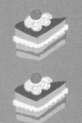 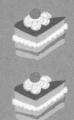 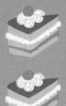 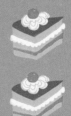

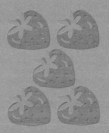 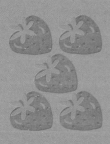 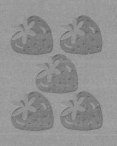

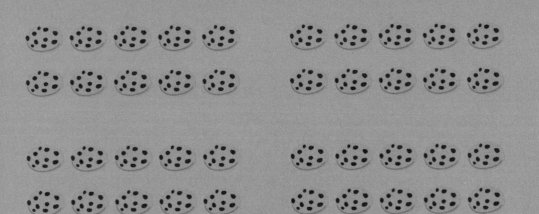

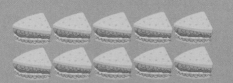 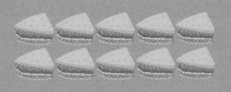 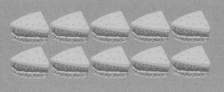

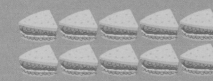 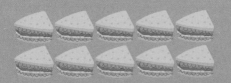

All Square

Create an array for each of the multiplication problems by shading in squares. One has been done to show you how.

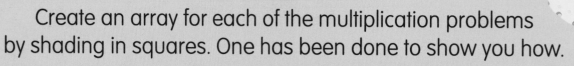

4 x 3 = 12

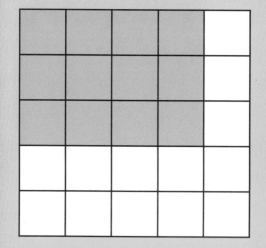

2 x 3 = 6

5 x 2 = 10

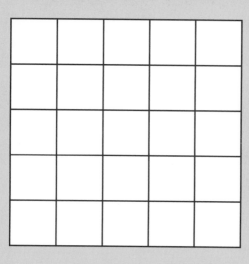

4 x 5 = 20

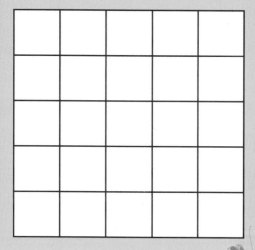

2 x 4 = 8

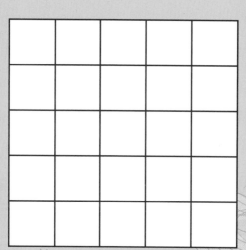

3 x 5 = 15

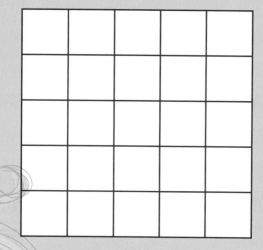

12

Castle Array

Add windows to each section of the castle,
like the example, to represent the
multiplication problems in the clouds.

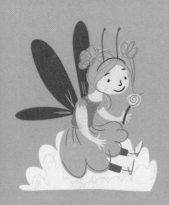

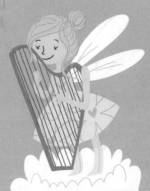

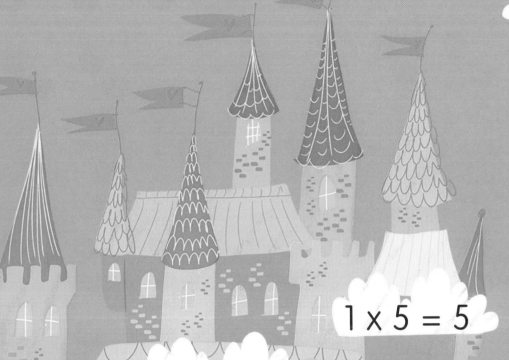

$1 \times 5 = 5$

$6 \times 3 = 18$

$2 \times 3 = 6$

$3 \times 3 = 9$

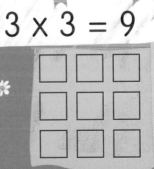

Double Trouble

Fairy Flo is picking cherries. Double the number of bunches to find how many cherries she picks each time.

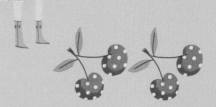

2 bunches = **4** cherries

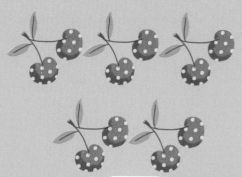

5 bunches = ☐ cherries

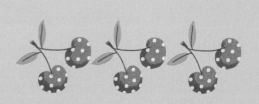

3 bunches = ☐ cherries

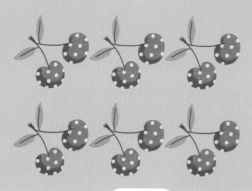

6 bunches = ☐ cherries

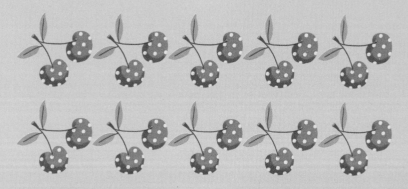

10 bunches = ☐ cherries

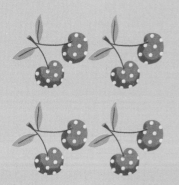

4 bunches = ☐ cherries

14

Sharing Is Fun

Tilly loves to grow flowers and give them to her friends.
She gives half of each set to Billy and Lily.
Draw round half of each group to work out the answer.

10 ÷ 2 = ☐

6 ÷ 2 = ☐

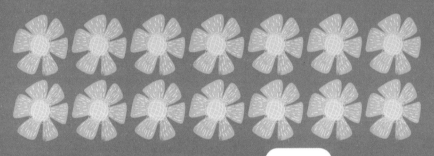

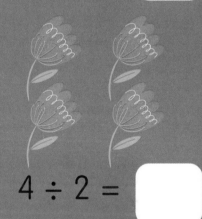

14 ÷ 2 = ☐

4 ÷ 2 = ☐

8 ÷ 2 = ☐

12 ÷ 2 = ☐

Ribbit!

There are five frogs and ten lily pads. Give each frog an equal number of unoccupied lily pads by sharing them and drawing round each group.

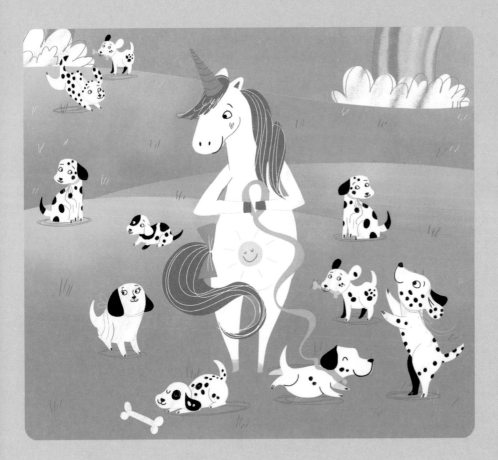

Spotted

Jasper is surrounded by cute puppies! Help him divide the spotty dogs into two groups of five, and five groups of two.

$$10 \div 2 = \boxed{}$$

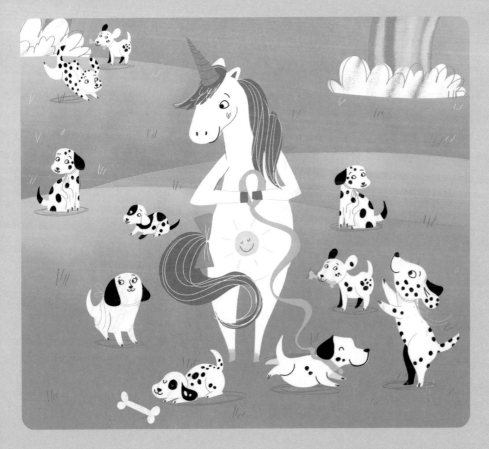

$$10 \div 5 = \boxed{}$$

Undersea Treasures

How many of each treasure will the creatures
have if they share the items in each group?

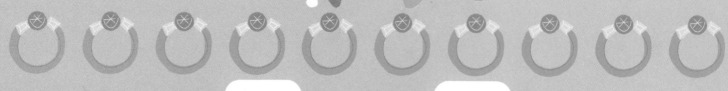

$$\boxed{} \div 2 = \boxed{}$$

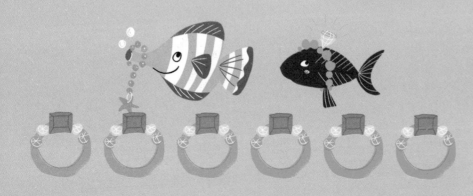

$$\boxed{} \div 2 = \boxed{}$$

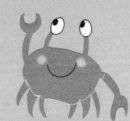

$$\boxed{} \div 2 = \boxed{}$$

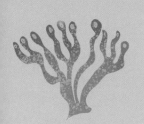
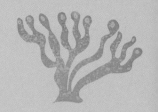

Merpeople Treasure

Now share out the jewels so the merpeople
and fairies have some, too!

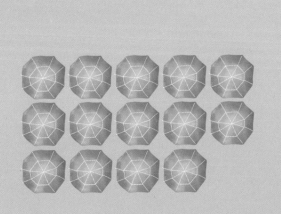
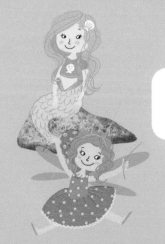

$\boxed{} \div 2 = \boxed{}$

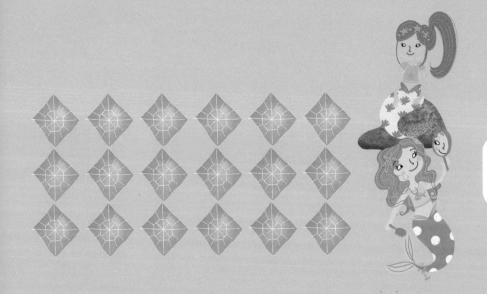
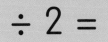

$\boxed{} \div 2 = \boxed{}$

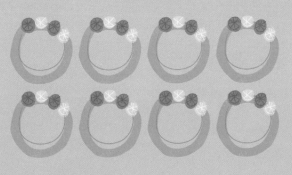
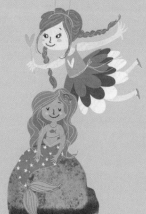

$\boxed{} \div 2 = \boxed{}$

Lighting the Night

The fireflies are gathering! If 2 more arrive every minute, how many will there be at the end?

1 x 2 =

2 x 2 =

3 x 2 =

4 x 2 =

5 x 2 =

6 x 2 =

7 x 2 =

8 x 2 =

9 x 2 =

10 x 2 =

11 x 2 =

12 x 2 =

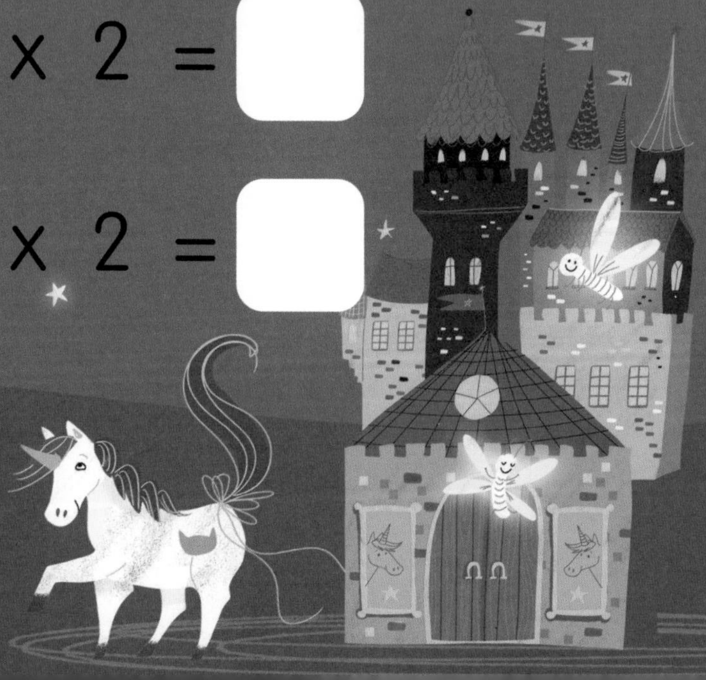

Heading for Home

Help the mermaid swim back to her father. She can only pass numbers that can be divided by two.

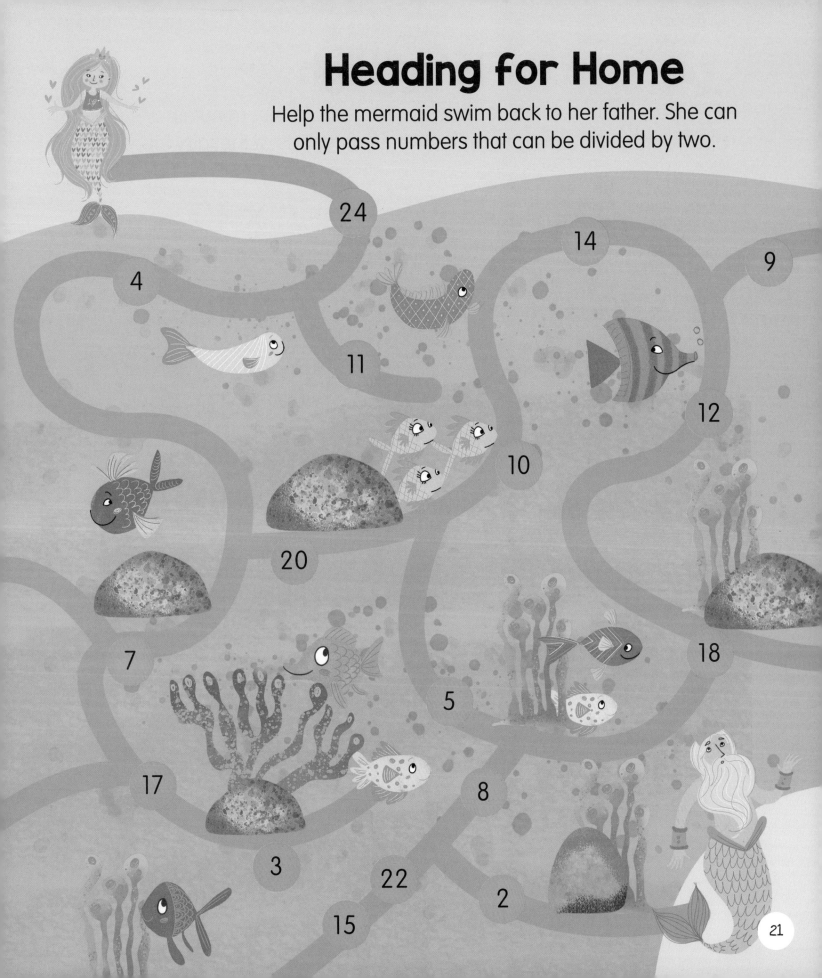

Flying High

Each of the fairies rides on Majestic for ten minutes.
How long is Majestic flying for if she carries lots of the fairy friends?

1 x 10 = ☐

2 x 10 = ☐

3 x 10 = ☐

4 x 10 = ☐

5 x 10 = ☐

6 x 10 = ☐

7 x 10 = ☐

8 x 10 = ☐

9 x 10 = ☐

10 x 10 = ☐

11 x 10 = ☐

12 x 10 = ☐

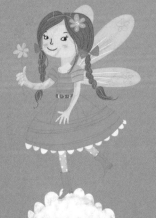
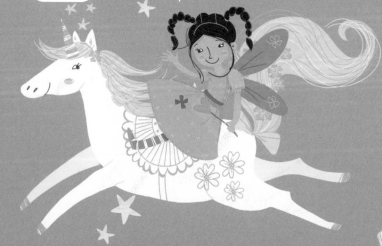
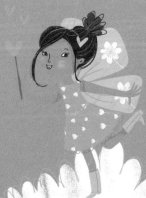

In the Circle

Help Sparklebreeze complete the division circle. Divide the inner numbers by ten, and write the answers in the outer circle.

The first one has been done for you.

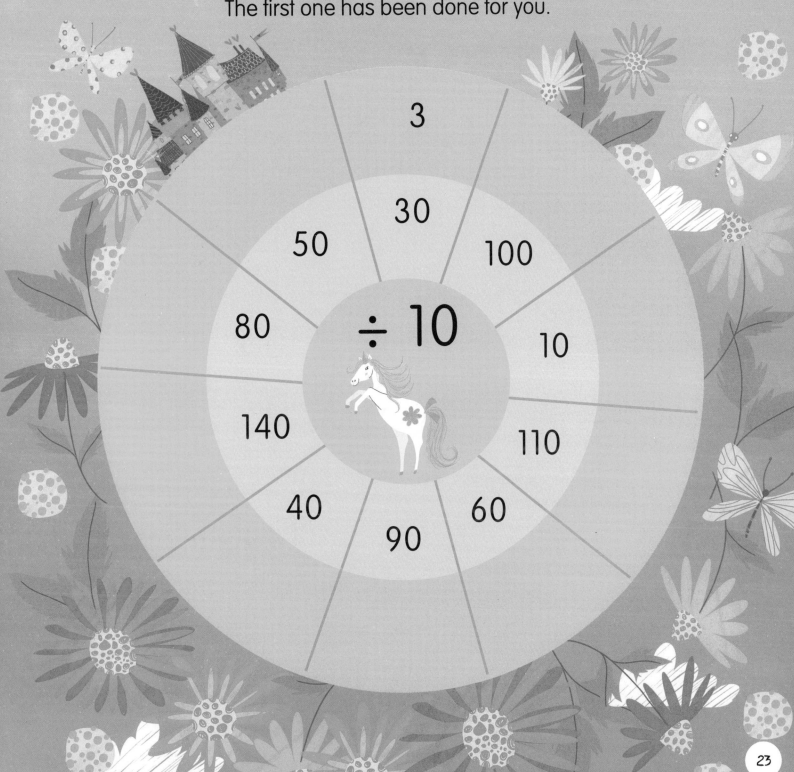

Inner circle numbers: 30, 100, 10, 110, 60, 90, 40, 140, 80, 50

Outer circle: 3 (÷ 10)

Fairy Fives

Can you help the five fairy friends complete the five times table?

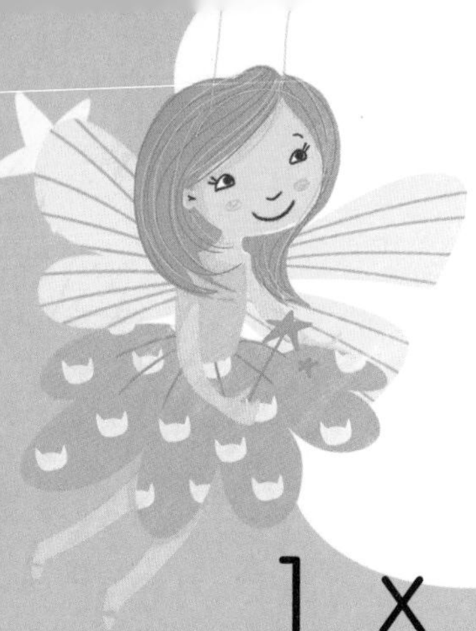

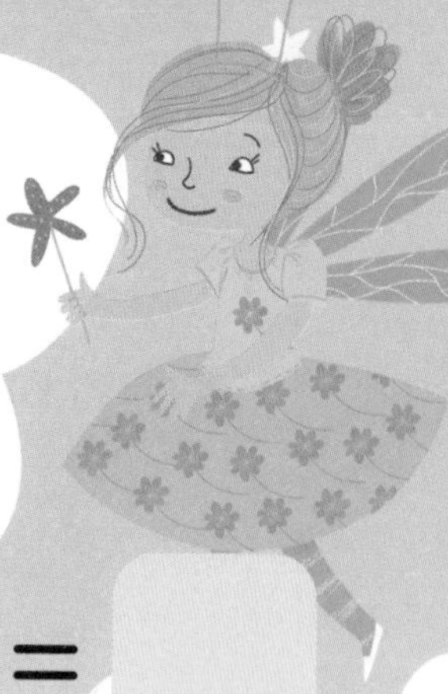

1 x 5 =

2 x 5 =

3 x 5 =

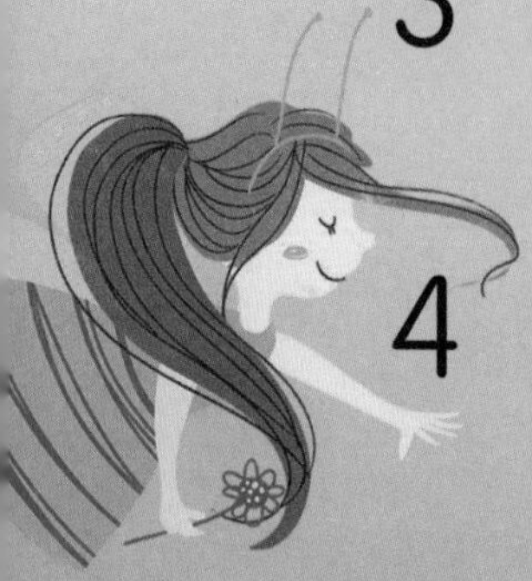

4 x 5 =

5 x 5 =

6 x 5 =

7 x 5 =

8 x 5 =

9 x 5 =

10 x 5 =

11 x 5 =

12 x 5 =

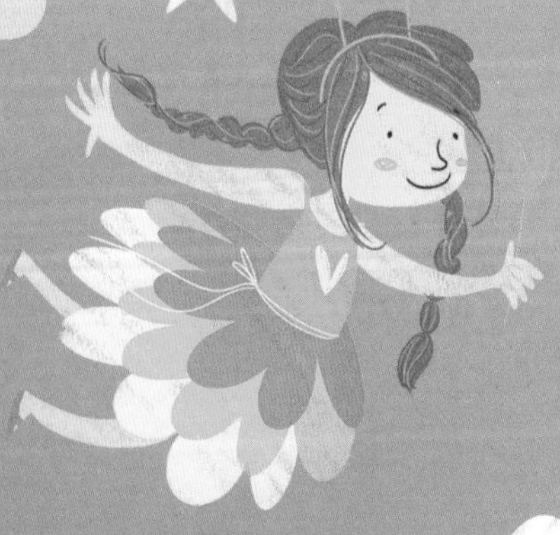

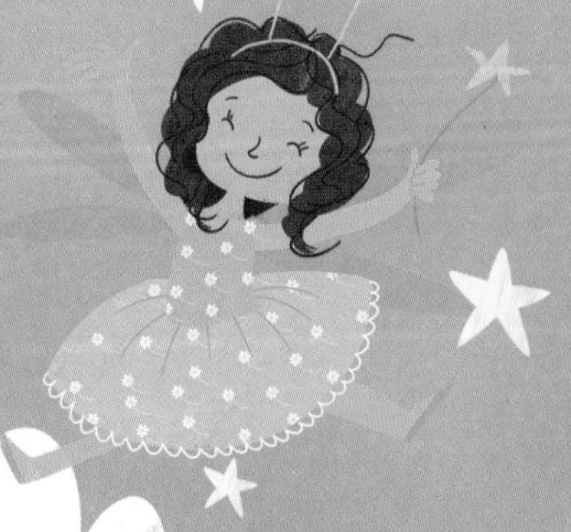

Give Me Five

The party friends need to find the answer that matches the problem on each of the baskets. Draw lines to link them up.

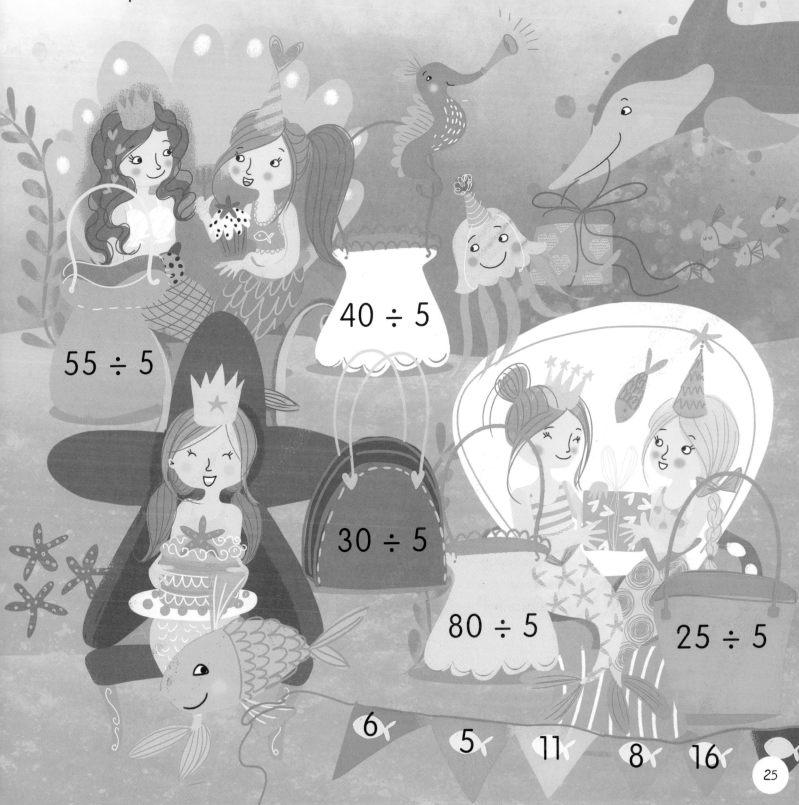

40 ÷ 5

55 ÷ 5

30 ÷ 5

80 ÷ 5

25 ÷ 5

6   5   11   8   16

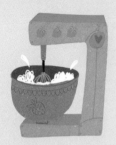

In the Kitchen

Help Fairy Clairey work out the
answers to these problems.

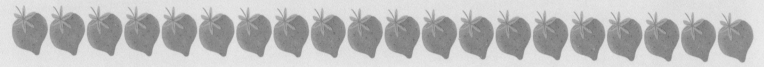

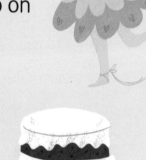

She has 20 strawberries. How many would go on
each cake if she decorates two cakes?

What about five cakes?

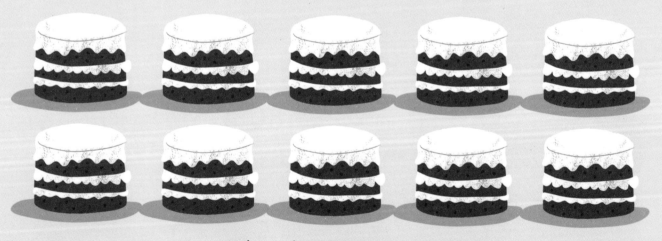

What about ten cakes?

Squirrel Away

Squirrel Harry has 20 acorns. He will hide them all away to see him through the winter.

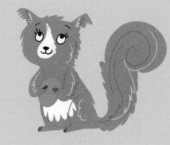

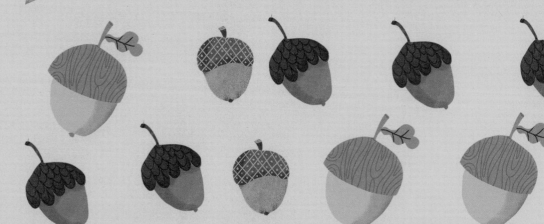

How many will there be if he divides them between two hiding places?

$20 \div 2 = \boxed{}$

How many will there be if he divides them between five hiding places?

$20 \div 5 = \boxed{}$

How many will there be if he divides them between ten hiding places?

$20 \div 10 = \boxed{}$

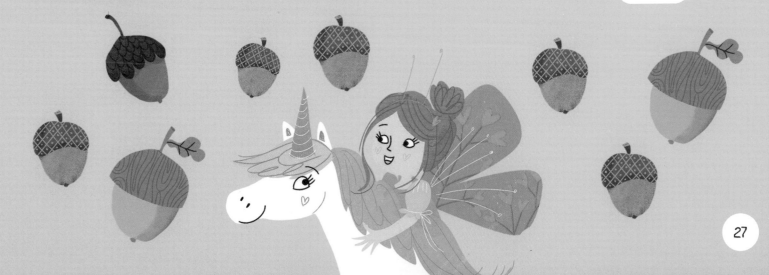

Thirsty Work

Granny Grimble drinks three cups
of tea every day. How many cups of tea
will she drink in a week? How many in 12 days?

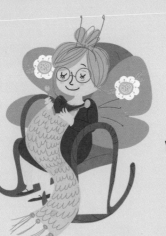

1 x 3 =

2 x 3 =

3 x 3 =

4 x 3 =

5 x 3 =

6 x 3 =

7 x 3 =

8 x 3 =

9 x 3 =

10 x 3 =

11 x 3 =

12 x 3 =

Threes in the Sea

Find a fish with the correct answer to each of these problems. They don't need to look the same each time.

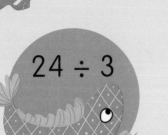

$24 \div 3$

$30 \div 3$

$36 \div 3$

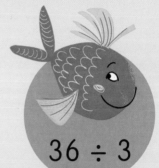

6

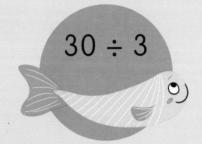

2

$12 \div 3$

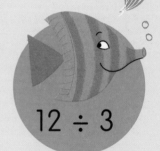

8

7

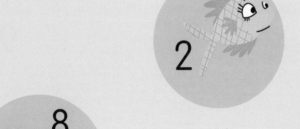

$18 \div 3$

12

4

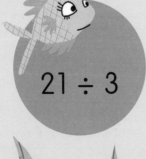

$21 \div 3$

10

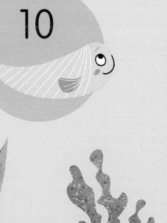

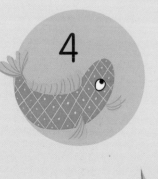

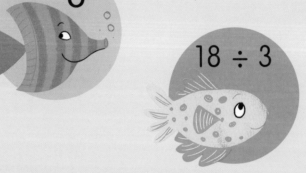

$6 \div 3$

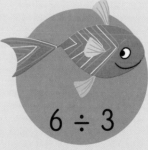

29

Wish on a Star

Spirit grants four wishes every day. How many wishes does she grant day after day?

1 x 4 =

2 x 4 =

3 x 4 =

4 x 4 =

5 x 4 =

6 x 4 =

7 x 4 =

8 x 4 =

9 x 4 =

10 x 4 =

11 x 4 =

12 x 4 =

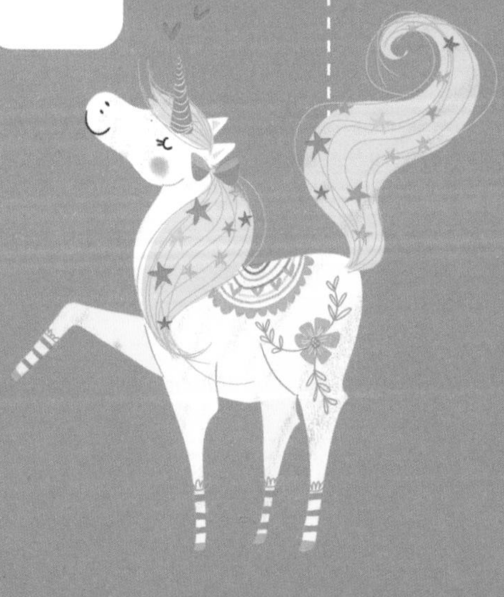

Hidden Treasure

Coral has found hidden treasure. How much will each of her family get if she divides it between the four of them?

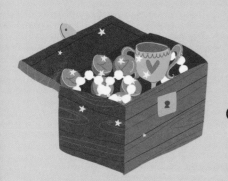

8 goblets	2	2	2	2
12 ruby rings				
4 diamonds				
16 bracelets				
20 brooches				
24 coins				

Whatever the Weather

The forecast predicts rain for six days every month.
How many days of rain are predicted through the year?

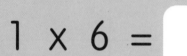

1 x 6 =

2 x 6 =

3 x 6 =

4 x 6 =

5 x 6 =

6 x 6 =

7 x 6 =

8 x 6 =

9 x 6 =

10 x 6 =

11 x 6 =

12 x 6 =

Factors With Six

Divide the top number by six and write the answer on the blank leaf. Ivy has done the first one to show you how.

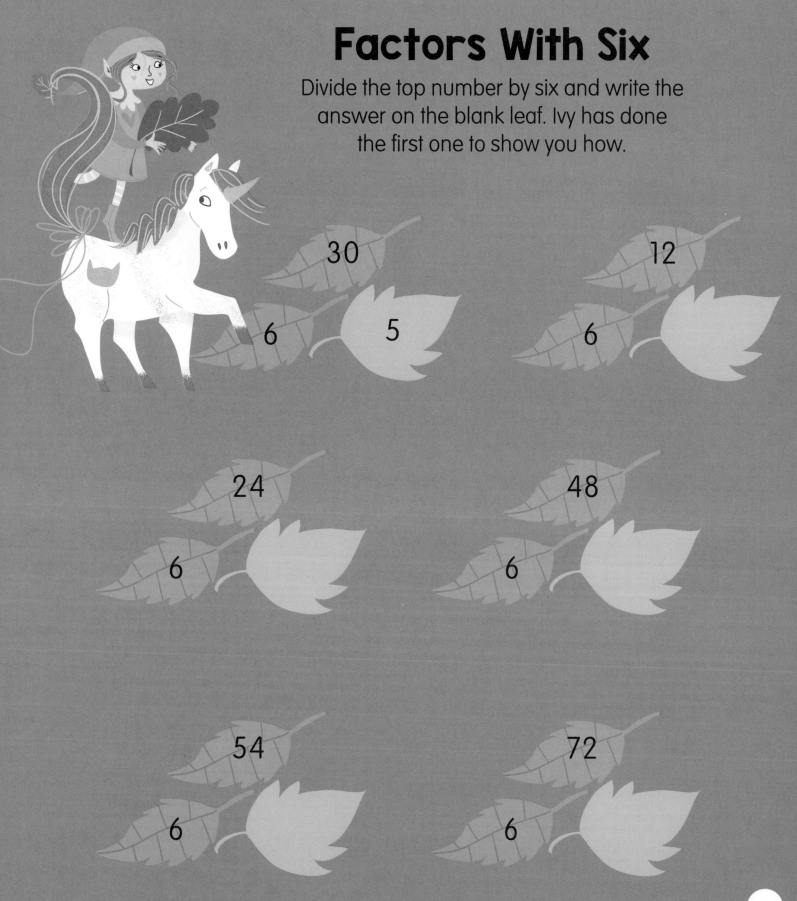

30
6
5

12
6

24
6

48
6

54
6

72
6

Visiting Friends

Connect each fairy to the castle that contains a multiple of their number. For example, fairy 4 can visit on any number that can be divided by 4, such as 12.

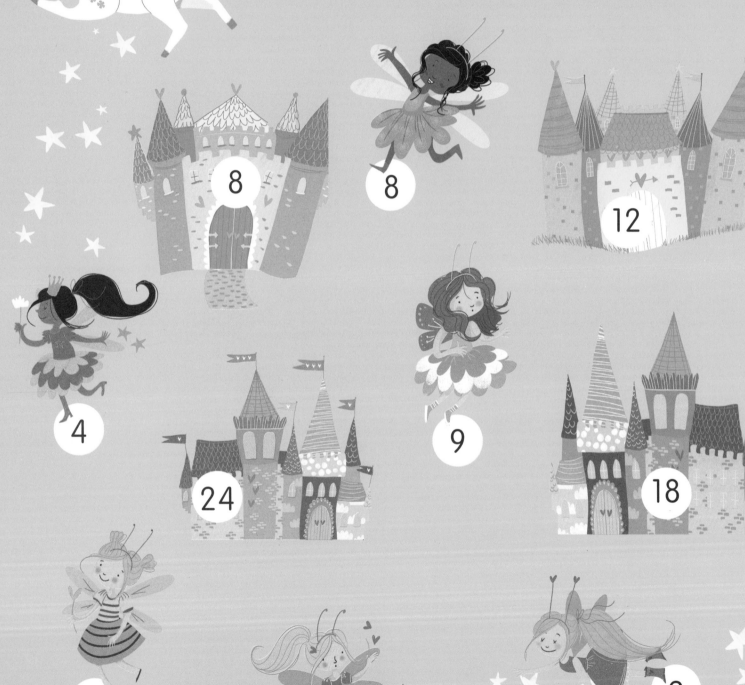

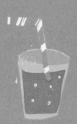
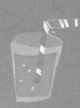

In the Kitchen

Freddy and Flossie have baked 24 cookies.
Can you help to share them among their friends?

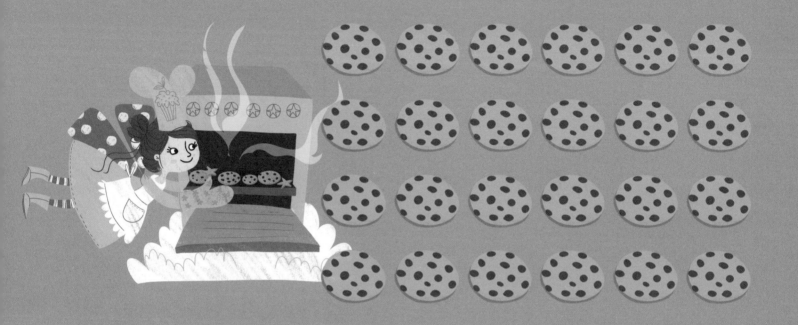

Share them between six friends.

Share them between four friends.

Share them between three friends.

Freddy and Flossie eat two cookies
each. If they give four friends the rest,
how many will each friend receive?

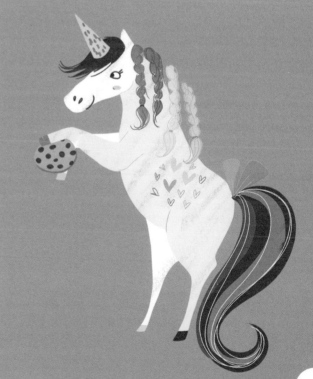

35

Wonderful Water

Tilly drinks a pitcher of water every day when it's hot.
How many pitchers does she drink through the weeks?

1 x 7 =

2 x 7 =

3 x 7 =

4 x 7 =

5 x 7 =

6 x 7 =

7 x 7 =

8 x 7 =

9 x 7 =

10 x 7 =

11 x 7 =

12 x 7 =

Seahorse Sevens

Match up pairs of seahorses so that each question has its correct answer.

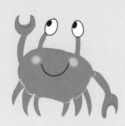

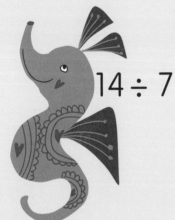

$14 \div 7$

3

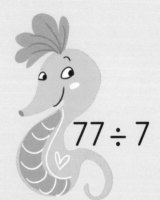

$77 \div 7$

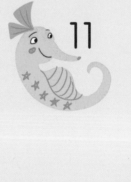

11

2

5

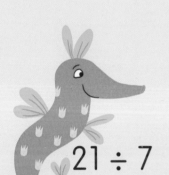

$21 \div 7$

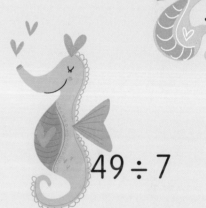

$49 \div 7$

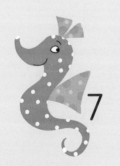

7

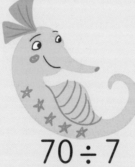

$70 \div 7$

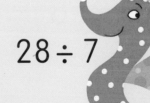

$28 \div 7$

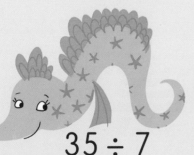

$35 \div 7$

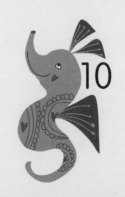

10

4

37

Fairy Rings

Eight new toadstools appear in the fairy grove every day.
How many toadstools appear after the number
of days shown below?

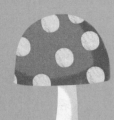
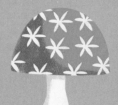

1 x 8 =

2 x 8 =

3 x 8 =

4 x 8 =

5 x 8 =

6 x 8 =

7 x 8 =

8 x 8 =

9 x 8 =

10 x 8 =

11 x 8 =

12 x 8 =

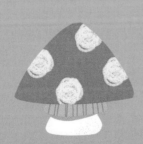
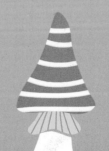

Eight Times Table

Divide each number in the lefthand grids by eight.
Write the answers in the righthand boxes. Skybreeze
and Snowflake have done the first ones to help you.

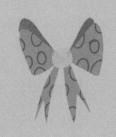

80	40	24
56	32	88
16	72	8
48	64	96

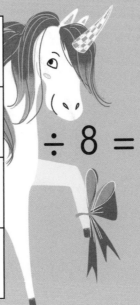

÷ 8 =

10	5	3

8	72	56
24	40	80
32	16	64
96	48	88

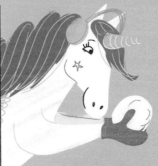

÷ 8 =

Beautiful Bunches

If each bouquet contains nine flowers,
how many flowers are in the number of bunches
written out below?

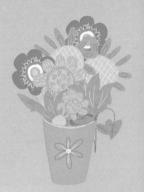

1 x 9 =

2 x 9 =

3 x 9 =

4 x 9 =

5 x 9 =

6 x 9 =

7 x 9 =

8 x 9 =

9 x 9 =

10 x 9 =

11 x 9 =

12 x 9 =

Sound Asleep

Shh! Don't wake the sleeping unicorns! Solve the problems as quickly and quietly as you can by dividing the inner numbers by nine.

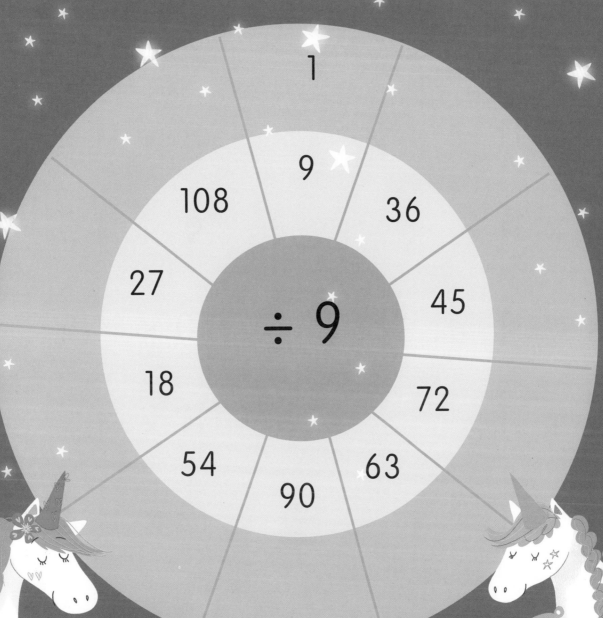

The first one has been done for you.

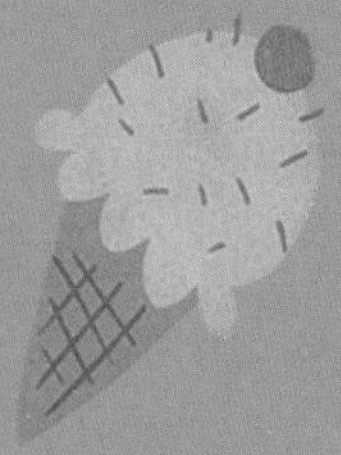

Days in the Sun

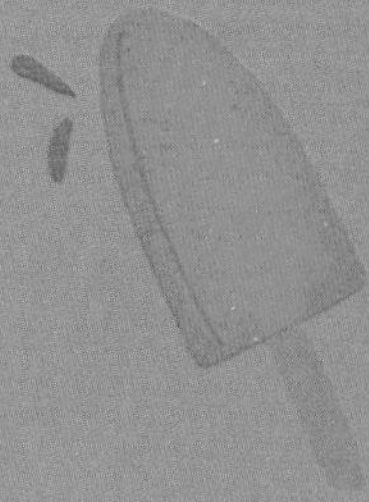

The ice cream fairy sells eleven items every hour. How many has she sold after the number of hours written out below?

1 x 11 =

2 x 11 =

3 x 11 =

4 x 11 =

5 x 11 =

6 x 11 =

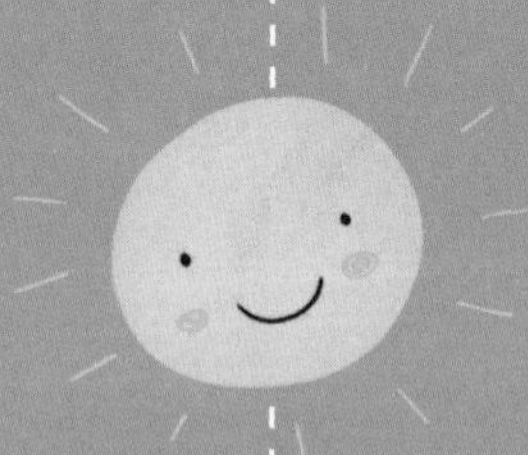

7 x 11 =

8 x 11 =

9 x 11 =

10 x 11 =

11 x 11 =

12 x 11 =

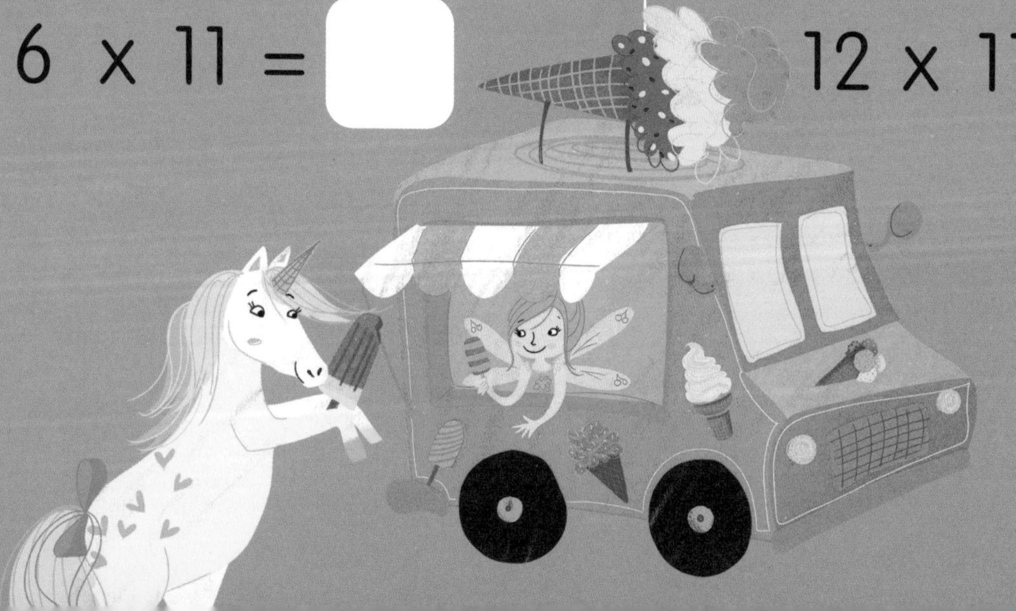

Spot It!

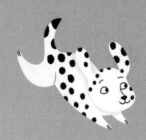

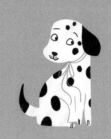

Each grid has one number that can't
be divided by 11. Can you spot it?

66	132	77
44	22	101
99	11	33
121	88	55

66	88	22
110	77	132
111	11	121
33	44	99

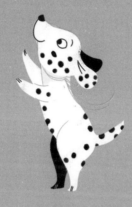

44	77	55
11	121	88
132	22	110
91	33	99

140	88	33
132	99	11
66	44	22
121	55	110

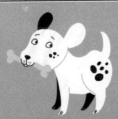

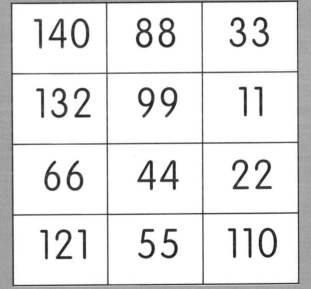

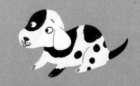

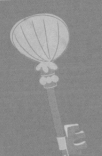

Happy Times

Sugar Sparkles visits her grandparents 12 times a month.
How many times does she visit them in
the number of months written out below?

1 x 12 =

2 x 12 =

3 x 12 =

4 x 12 =

5 x 12 =

6 x 12 =

7 x 12 =

8 x 12 =

9 x 12 =

10 x 12 =

11 x 12 =

12 x 12 =

Sweet Music

Circle the musical notes that do not have multiples of 12. How many are there?

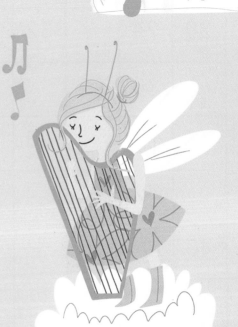

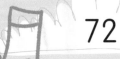
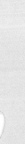
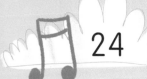

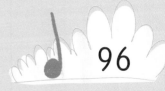
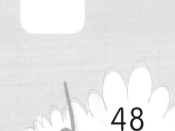

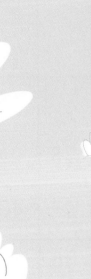
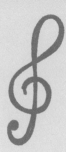
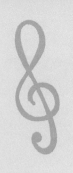
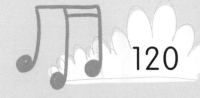

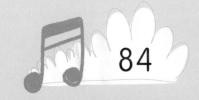
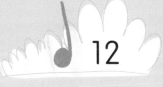
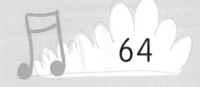

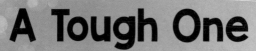

A Tough One

Multiply the numbers in the blue row by the numbers in the blue column to fill in the answers in the grid.

1	2	3	4	5	6	7	8	9	10	11	12
2			8			14	16		20	22	
3	6					21		27		33	
4		12		20	24		32		40		48
5	10	15			30	35		45			
6	12	18					48			66	72
7			28		42			63			84
8		24		40		56			80		
9	18		36		54		72			99	108
10		30		50		70		90		110	120
11			44	55	66	77	88				
12	24	36		60			96			132	

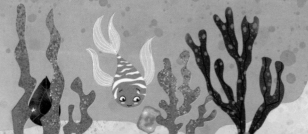

Fairy Factors

Flossie has a selection of factors for each of her numbers.
One of them is wrong in each group—can you spot it?

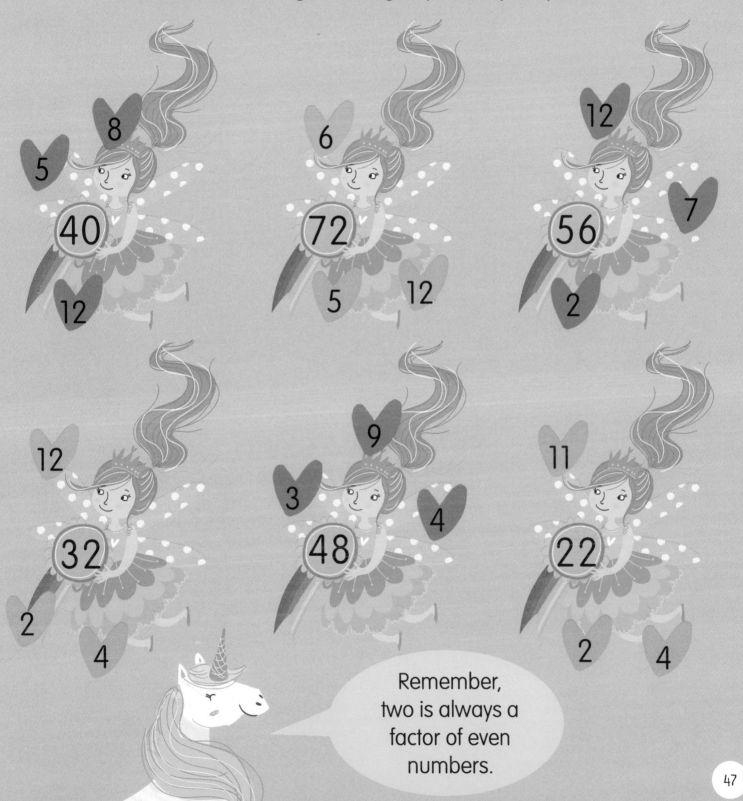

Remember,
two is always a
factor of even
numbers.

Daisy Chains

Which of the numbers on each daisy chain are not factors of the number on the leaf?

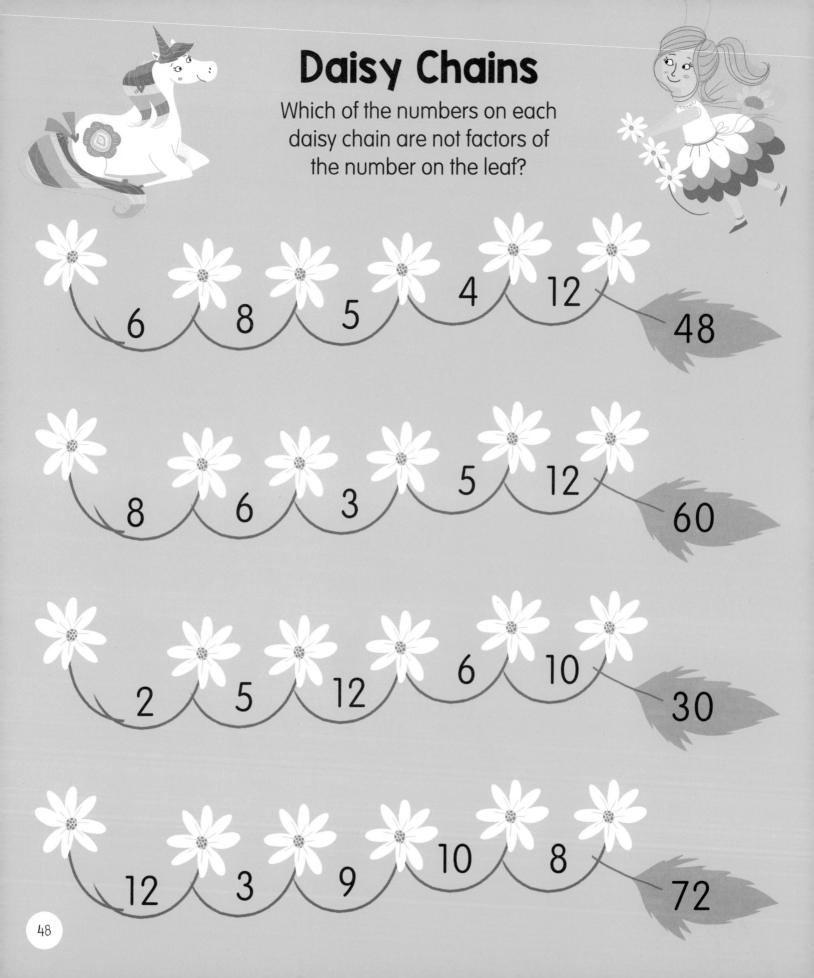

6   8   5   4   12   **48**

8   6   3   5   12   **60**

2   5   12   6   10   **30**

12   3   9   10   8   **72**

Feeling Crabby

Fill in the gaps so each crab's two numbers multiply to make the number in the star.

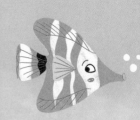

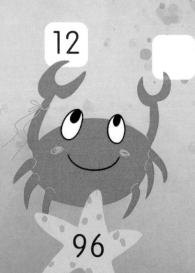

12 · ☐

96

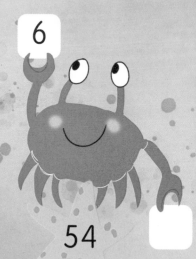

6 · ☐

54

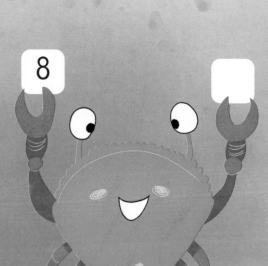

8 · ☐

48

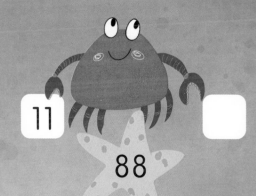

11 · ☐

88

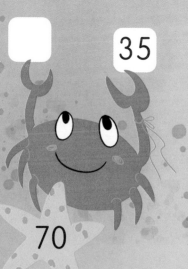

☐ · 35

70

Octo-Puzzler

Each octopus has a factor number.
Which of the rocks can each hide behind?

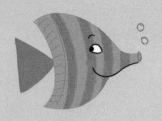

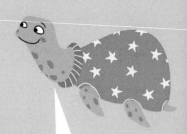

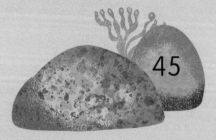

All numbers are factors of themselves.

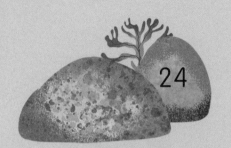

24

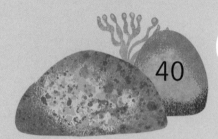

40

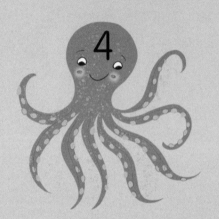

4

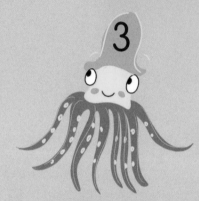

3

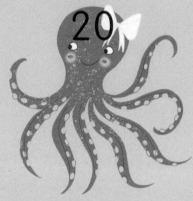

20

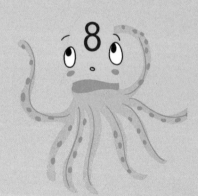

8

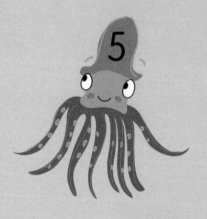

5

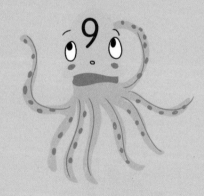

9

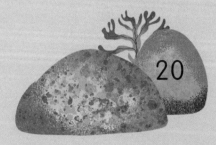

20

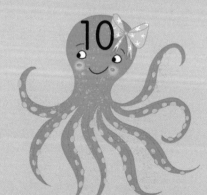

10

45

50

A Thing of Beauty

There are 24 butterflies in the garden.
They fly off and land on the bushes. Work out
how many there are in each scenario.

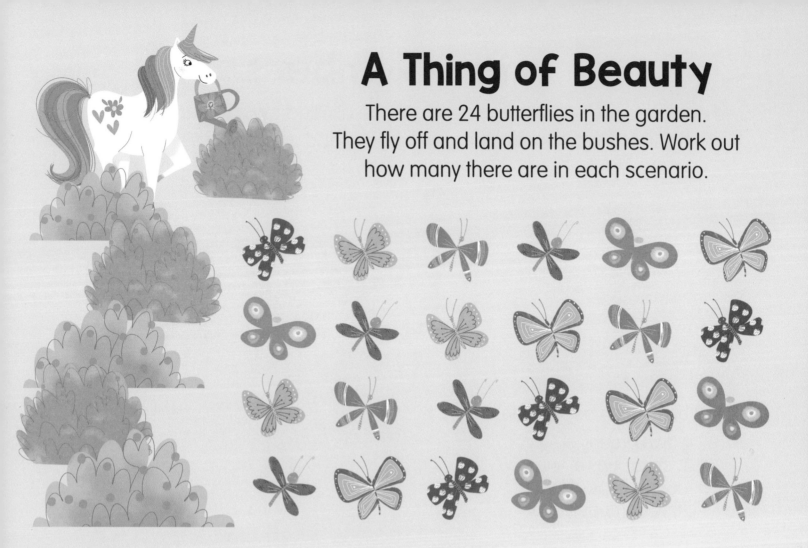

How many will there be on each bush, if an
equal number land on each of six bushes?

How many will there be on each bush, if an
equal number land on each of four bushes?

How many will there be on each bush, if an
equal number land on each of three bushes?

Six more butterflies appear! Now how many are
there if they land in equal numbers on six bushes?

Prime Numbers

Prime numbers are special. They can only be divided by themselves, and by one.
Which of these groups of blocks can't be divided into smaller equal groups?

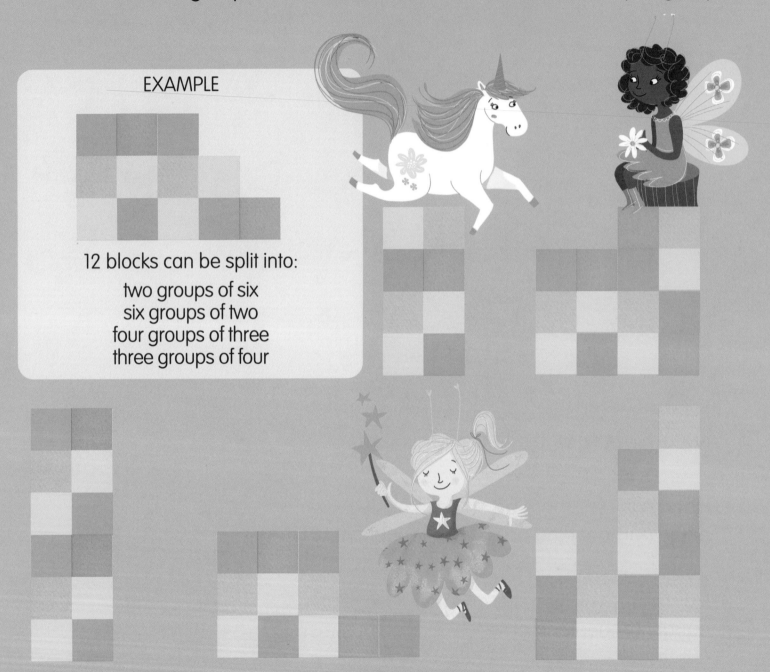

EXAMPLE

12 blocks can be split into:

two groups of six
six groups of two
four groups of three
three groups of four

Write all the prime numbers under 20 that you can think of.

52

In the Air

Use the clues to work out which balloon belongs to each of the unicorns.

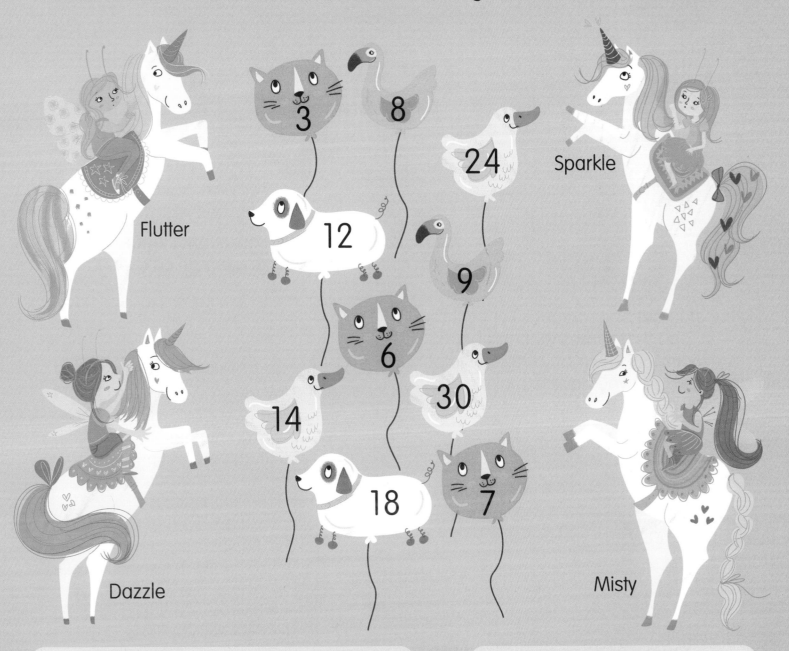

Flutter

Sparkle

Dazzle

Misty

3 8 24 12 9 6 14 30 18 7

Dazzle's balloon is a prime number lower than 10 but higher than 5.

Sparkle's balloon is a multiple of 9 and also of 6.

Flutter's balloon is the highest common factor of 48 and 72.

Misty's balloon can only be divided by 7 and 2.

Scaling Solutions

Baking in bulk can be tricky.
Can you solve these problems?

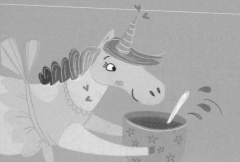
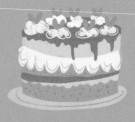

You get an order for 10 chocolate and three times that number of vanilla. How many cakes in total do you have to make?

If you can bake 24 cakes in an hour, how many can you bake in 3 hours?

You decorate each vanilla cake with two cherries. How many cherries will 80 cakes need?

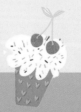

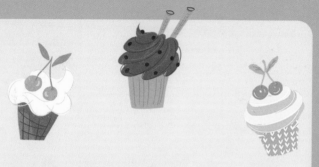

You make 100 rainbow cakes and half that amount of lemon cakes. How many lemon cakes is that?

Chocolate cakes sell three times as many as strawberry. You sell 15 strawberry cupcakes in an hour. How many chocolate do you sell in the same time?

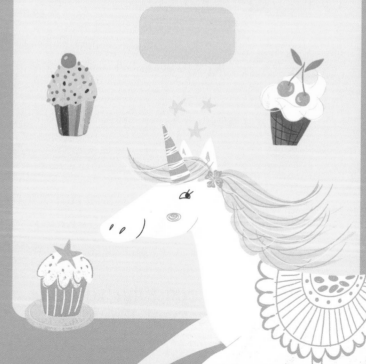

54

Bird Watching

The unicorns love to watch out for birds in the garden.
Help them with the multiplication problems here.

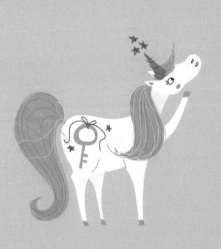
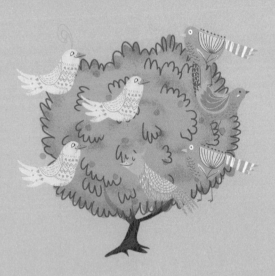
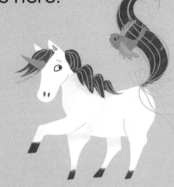

If the same birds are in the tree every day for 2 days, how many of
each type of bird will they have seen?

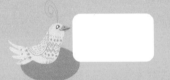 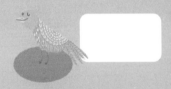 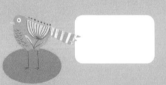 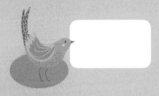

If the same birds are in the tree every day for 4 days, how many of
each type of bird will they have seen?

 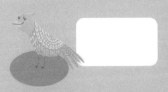 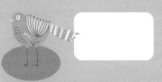 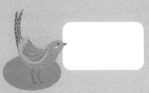

If the same birds are in the tree every day for a week, how many of
each type of bird will they have seen?

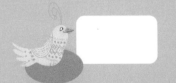 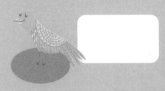 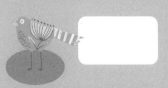 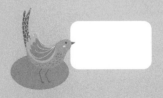

Festive Fun

Fill in the missing numbers and then celebrate!

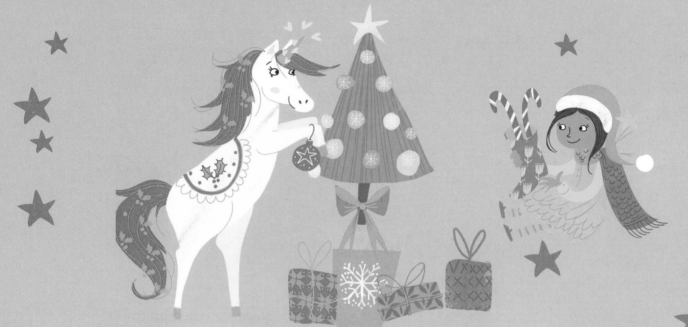

8 x ☐ = 40   32 ÷ ☐ = 8

☐ x 9 = 99   ☐ ÷ 9 = 4

9 x ☐ = 18   60 ÷ ☐ = 5

☐ x 7 = 49   ☐ ÷ 8 = 2

6 x ☐ = 24   55 ÷ ☐ = 5

Hide and Seek

Fill in the missing signs to make these problems work properly. The hiding fairies might help you!

$2 \boxed{\times} 7 = 14$

$24 \boxed{} 3 = 8$

$8 \boxed{\times} 8 = 64$

$7 \boxed{} 5 = 35$

$54 \boxed{} 9 = 6$

$63 \boxed{} 9 = 7$

$28 \boxed{} 4 = 7$

$12 \boxed{} 2 = 6$

$49 \boxed{} 7 = 7$

$6 \boxed{} 3 = 18$

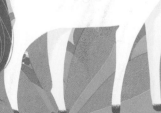

Whoops!

The mermaids have got some of these problems wrong.
Can you spot three mistakes, and make them right?

$9 \times 7 = 56$

$8 \times 5 = 40$

$6 \times 6 = 36$

$11 \times 6 = 66$

$12 \times 2 = 22$

$4 \times 8 = 38$

$6 \times 7 = 42$

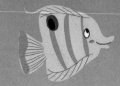

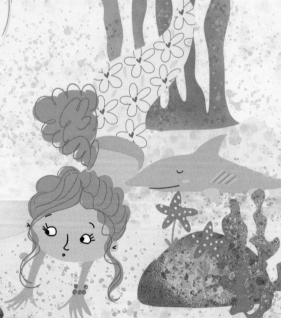

Coral Calculations

This coral reef is flourishing! Read the problems and work out the answers.

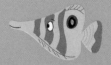

There are 88 fish on the reef.
If there are 11 fish in each shoal,
how many shoals are there?

Some of the fish lay eggs. Not all
of the eggs hatch. If 6 fish each
have 12 hatched eggs, how many
baby fish are there?

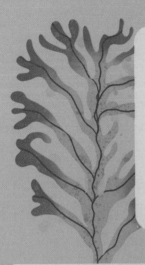

If each of the 8 shoals has 4 new
babies, how many new fish are
there in total?

Five of the fish gather shells.
If each fish collects 8 shells,
how many shells are there?

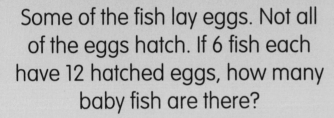
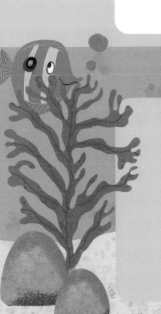
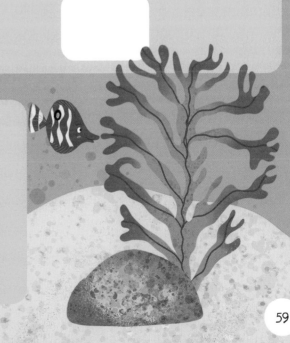

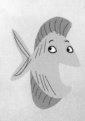
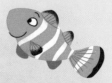

One to One

Experiment with multiplying and dividing by one.
The first set of answers will help you with the second set.

4 x 1 = ☐   8 x 1 = ☐

10 x 1 = ☐   20 x 1 = ☐

5 x 1 = ☐   50 x 1 = ☐

4 ÷ 1 = ☐   20 ÷ 1 = ☐

8 ÷ 1 = ☐   15 ÷ 1 = ☐

5 ÷ 1 = ☐   50 ÷ 1 = ☐

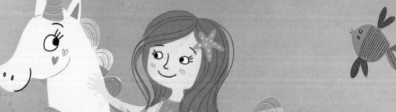

Zero Zone

Do you know what happens when you multiply by zero? It's easy, really, as the answer is always zero. Check it out with these calculations.

$9 \times 0 =$ ☐ $12 \times 0 =$ ☐

$40 \times 0 =$ ☐ $60 \times 0 =$ ☐

$90 \times 0 =$ ☐ $100 \times 0 =$ ☐

Now, let's try a really big number!

$5,000,000 \times 0 =$ ☐

What happens if you multiply a trillion by zero?
Write your answer in the box.

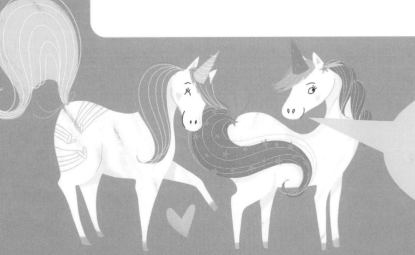

You can't divide a number by 0. Try sharing two sweets between nobody!

Cutie Pies

Help the animals fill in the grid by multiplying by ten each time.

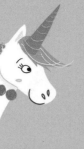
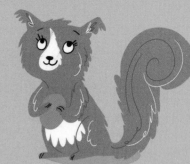

x 10	Hundreds	Tens	Units
2			
20			
6			
11			
16			
4			
18			
33			
88			

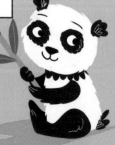
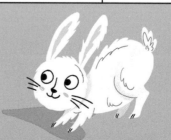
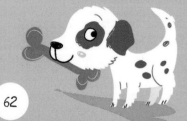
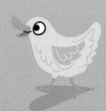

Mathematical Mirrors

Divide the lefthand numbers by ten, and write the answers in the mirrors on the righthand side, like the first example.

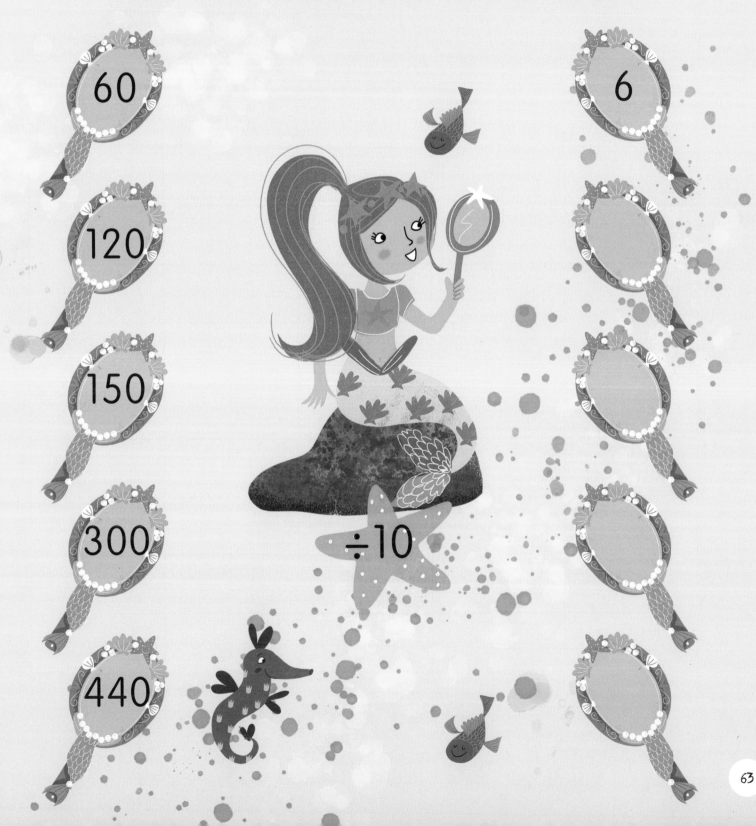

60

120

150

300

440

÷10

6

The Hundreds Table

Multiply the lefthand numbers by 100 to fill in all of the columns.

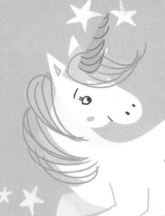

x 100	Thousands	Hundreds	Tens	Units
1				
20				
5				
18				
33				
9				
12				
66				
88				

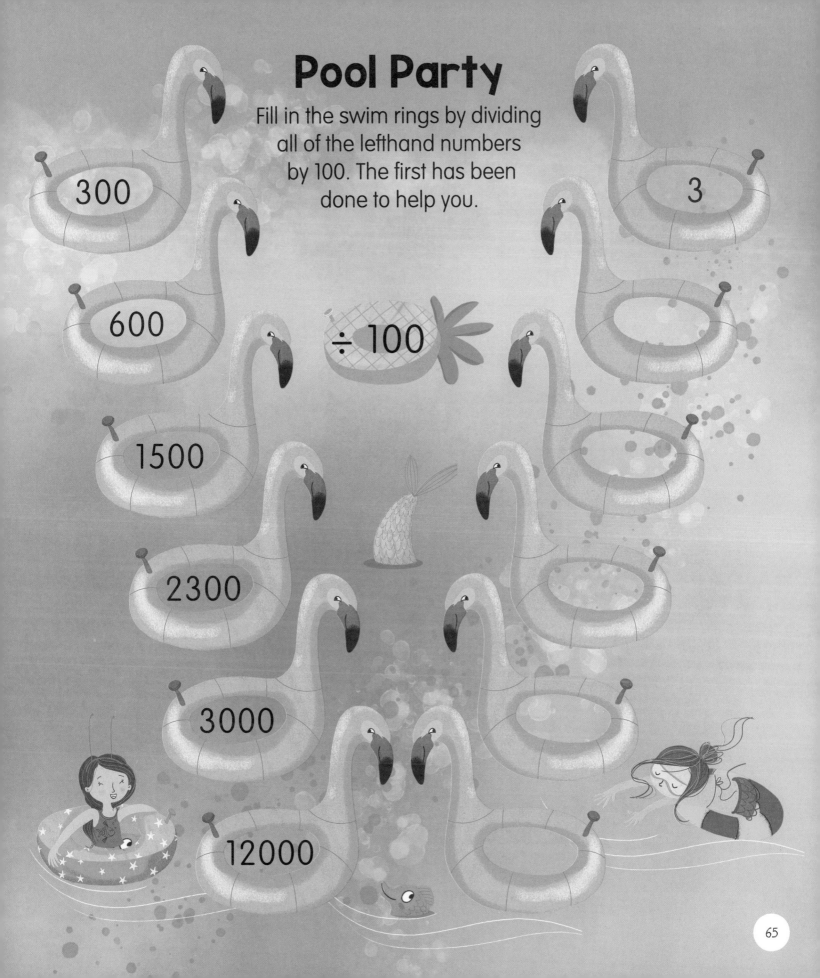

Pool Party

Fill in the swim rings by dividing all of the lefthand numbers by 100. The first has been done to help you.

300

3

600

÷ 100

1500

2300

3000

12000

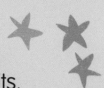

Superstars

Study the example to see how to use a grid to multiply two digits.
Multiply the tens first, and then the units, and add them together.

35 x 2

x	30	5
2	60	10

60 + 10 = 70

28 x 5

x	20	8
5		

☐ + ☐ = ☐

13 x 2

x	10	3
2		

☐ + ☐ = ☐

80 x 3

x	80	0
3		

☐ + ☐ = ☐

19 x 5

x	10	9
5		

☐ + ☐ = ☐

Tough Task

Once you have mastered the grid method,
fill in these grids and do the addition in your head.

14 x 4

x		

27 x 5

x		

19 x 6

x		

43 x 4

x		

38 x 8

x		

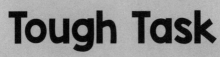

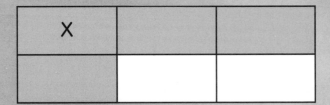

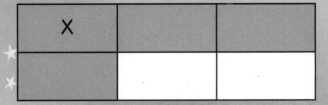

Logic Task

Multiply the units together in each problem. It will tell you the last digit, and help you guess which of the answers is correct.

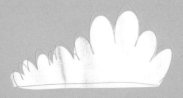
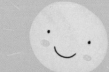

6 x 3 = 18, so the last digit must be 8!

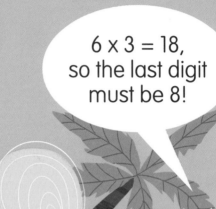

76 x 3   210

33 x 7   228

56 x 2   231

63 x 3   112

42 x 5   189

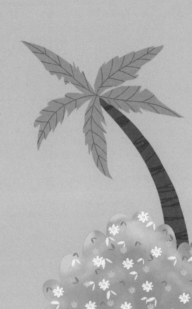

Now work them out in full, to check if you were right!

33 x 7

x	30	3
7		

56 x 2

x	50	6
2		

63 x 3

x	60	3
3		

42 x 5

x	40	2
5		

Taking Flight

Let the owl help you with a different method. Imagine it flying in two stages for each problem, like the example.

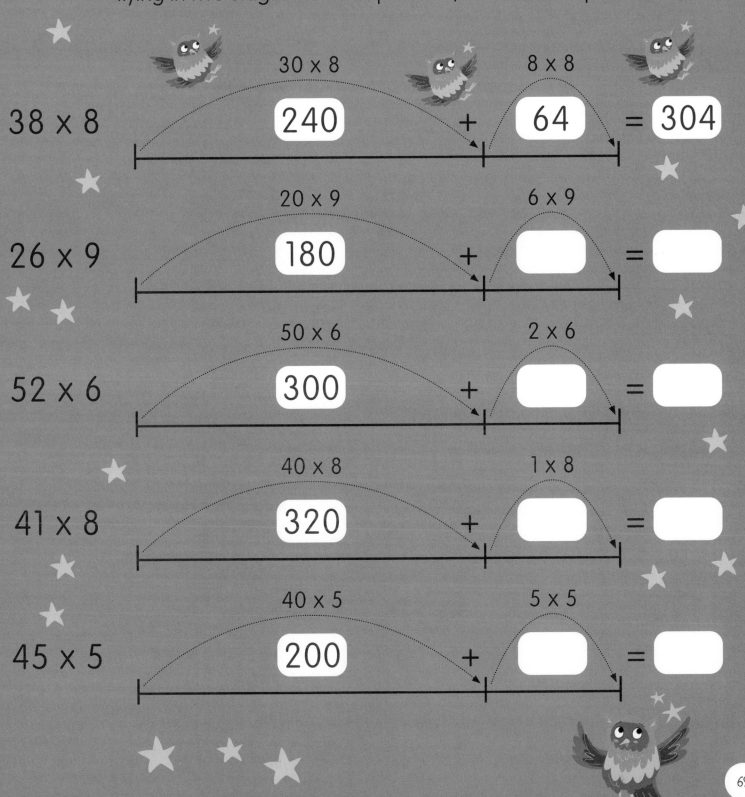

38 x 8

30 x 8 → 240 + 8 x 8 → 64 = 304

26 x 9

20 x 9 → 180 + 6 x 9 → ☐ = ☐

52 x 6

50 x 6 → 300 + 2 x 6 → ☐ = ☐

41 x 8

40 x 8 → 320 + 1 x 8 → ☐ = ☐

45 x 5

40 x 5 → 200 + 5 x 5 → ☐ = ☐

Something New

Here is another method. Multiply the units and carry over any tens.
Do the same with the numbers in the tens column.
Be careful with your columns! Add any numbers you
have carried over to get the final answer.

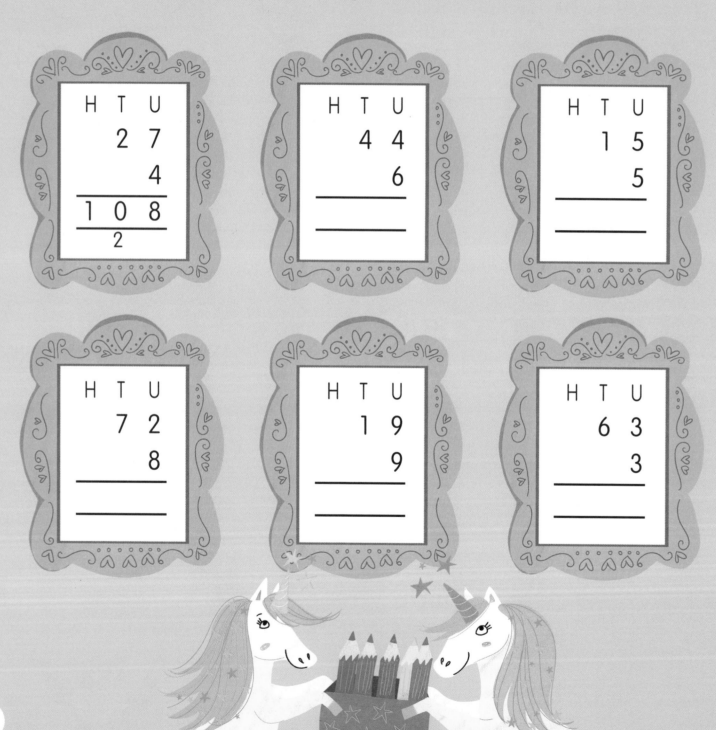

```
  H T U
    2 7
      4
  ─────
  1 0 8
    2
```

```
  H T U
    4 4
      6
  ─────
```

```
  H T U
    1 5
      5
  ─────
```

```
  H T U
    7 2
      8
  ─────
```

```
  H T U
    1 9
      9
  ─────
```

```
  H T U
    6 3
      3
  ─────
```

The Tea Room

Fairy Freya's tea room is very popular! Each of her large teapots holds seven cups of tea. Work out how many cups she served in the last week.

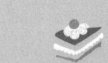

	Pots of tea	Total cups (seven per pot)
Monday	12	
Tuesday	16	
Wednesday	27	
Thursday	15	
Friday	34	
Saturday	39	
Sunday	29	

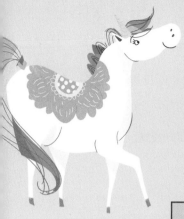

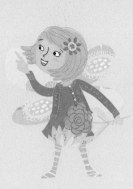

You Can Do It!

Use the grid method to multiply three digits.
Multiply the hundreds, then the tens, then the units,
and add them all together, like the example.

154 x 3

X	100	50	4
3	300	150	12

462

128 x 4

X			

316 x 5

X			

247 x 2

X			

565 x 3

X			

Do It Again!

Now use the column method to multiply three digits. Multiply the units, carrying over any tens, and repeat with the tens and hundreds. Be sure you get the numbers in the correct columns.

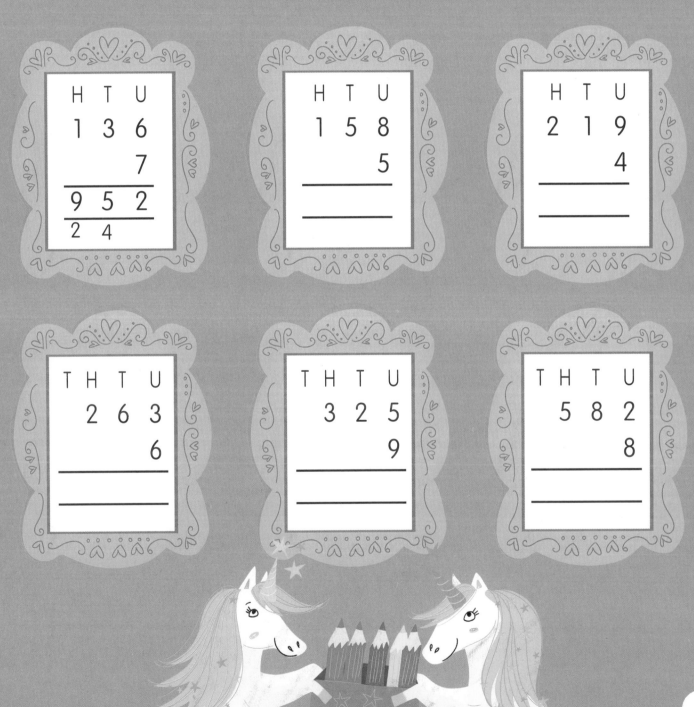

```
  H T U
  1 3 6
×     7
-------
  9 5 2
  2 4
```

```
  H T U
  1 5 8
×     5
-------

```

```
  H T U
  2 1 9
×     4
-------

```

```
TH T U
 2 6 3
×    6
------

```

```
TH T U
 3 2 5
×    9
------

```

```
TH T U
 5 8 2
×    8
------

```

Double Check

Use one method to work out the answers, then use
a different method to check you got them right.

	Answer	Check
19 x 6		
28 x 4		
35 x 9		
14 x 8		
44 x 7		

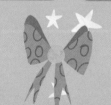

Check Again!

Here are some more for you to solve and then double check.

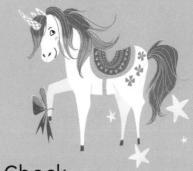

	Answer	Check
652 x 3		
271 x 6		
107 x 5		
348 x 2		
427 x 7		

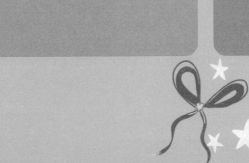

Fairy Facts

Each fairy has three numbers in her basket. Fill in the multiplication and division facts for each one. Use the example to help you.

7	x	5	=	35
5	x	7	=	35
35	÷	5	=	7
35	÷	7	=	5

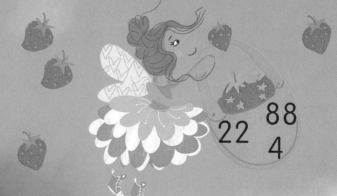

88
22
4

	x		=	
	x		=	
	÷		=	
	÷		=	

35
5
7

64 16
4

33 99
3

	x		=	
	x		=	
	÷		=	
	÷		=	

	x		=	
	x		=	
	÷		=	
	÷		=	

Work It Out

Follow the example using inverse relationships. When you know a multiplication fact, you can use it to work out two division facts.

$13 \times 7 = 91$

$91 \div 13 = 7$

$91 \div 7 = 13$

$24 \times 3 = 72$

$72 \div \boxed{} = \boxed{}$

$72 \div \boxed{} = \boxed{}$

$18 \times 5 = 90$

$\boxed{} \div \boxed{} = \boxed{}$

$\boxed{} \div \boxed{} = \boxed{}$

$16 \times 4 = 64$

$\boxed{} \div \boxed{} = \boxed{}$

$\boxed{} \div \boxed{} = \boxed{}$

Festive Fun

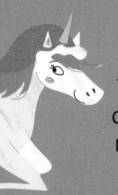

The unicorns are decorating six Christmas trees. How many of each type of ornament will go on each tree? Work out how many of each type there are, then divide that number by six. Will there be any left over?

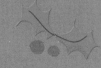

	Decorations bought	Working out	Left over
	5 packs of 10	5 x 10 = 50 6 x 8 is 48 so 50 ÷ 6 = 8 with 2 left over	2
	2 packs of 6		
	5 packs of 3		
	6 packs of 8		
	2 packs of 12		
	1 pack of 15		
	4 packs of 5		

Delicious!

Look at all these treats! Answer the questions
below to work out how to share them among friends.

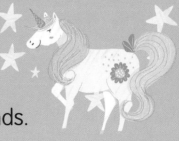

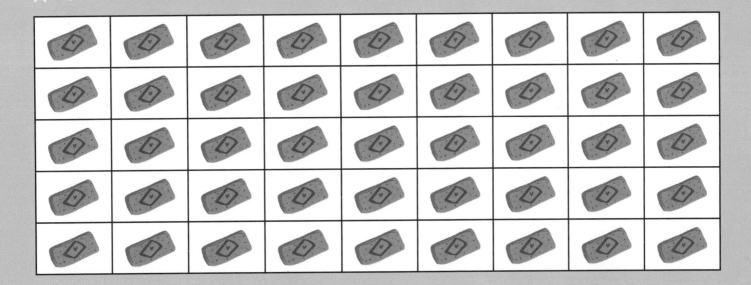

If the five unicorns share them equally,
how many would each unicorn have?

The unicorns decide to share with
another friend. To share them equally
between six, how many would each
unicorn have, ignoring remainders?

For how many days could they each
eat two per day?

How many do you need to cut in
half so all six have an equal share
of the remaining cookies?

If the five unicorns decide to each
eat three treats a day, how many
days would they last?

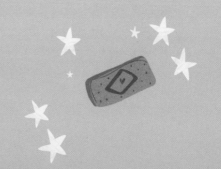

Dividing Made Easy

Use partitioning to help you divide—split the number into chunks, using the ten times table for the first part. Then divide the remainder. Don't forget to add the chunks together! The first one has been done for you.

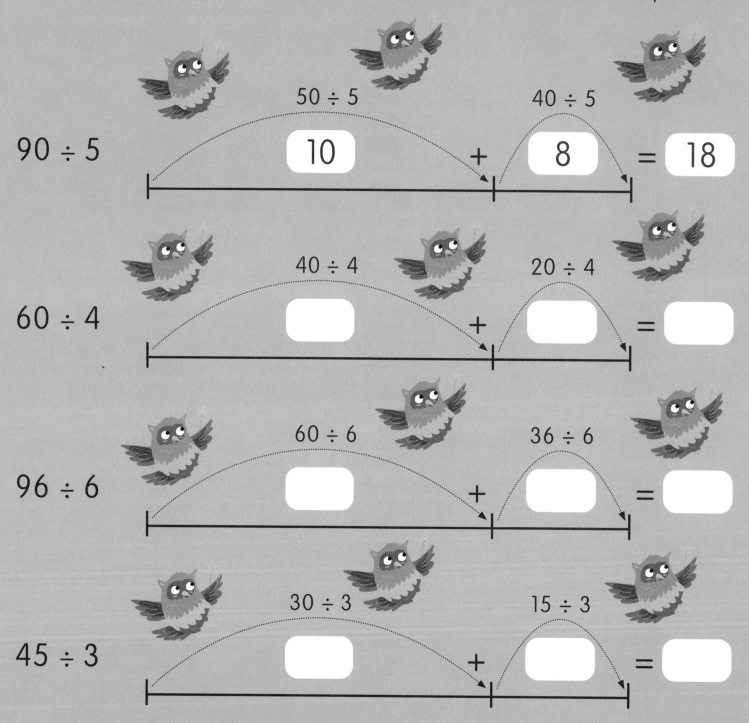

$90 \div 5$

$50 \div 5$ [10] + $40 \div 5$ [8] = [18]

$60 \div 4$

$40 \div 4$ [ ] + $20 \div 4$ [ ] = [ ]

$96 \div 6$

$60 \div 6$ [ ] + $36 \div 6$ [ ] = [ ]

$45 \div 3$

$30 \div 3$ [ ] + $15 \div 3$ [ ] = [ ]

Dividing Bigger Numbers

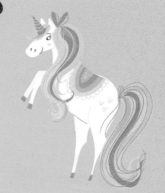

Now use the grid method to solve these.
Divide the tens first, and then the
remainder, like in the example.

85 ÷ 5

	10	7
5	50	35

10 + 7 = 17

38 ÷ 2

	10	9
2	20	18

10 + 9 =

96 ÷ 6

	10	
6		

10 + [ ] = [ ]

57 ÷ 3

	10	
3		

10 + [ ] = [ ]

More Division

Use these extra problems for practice.

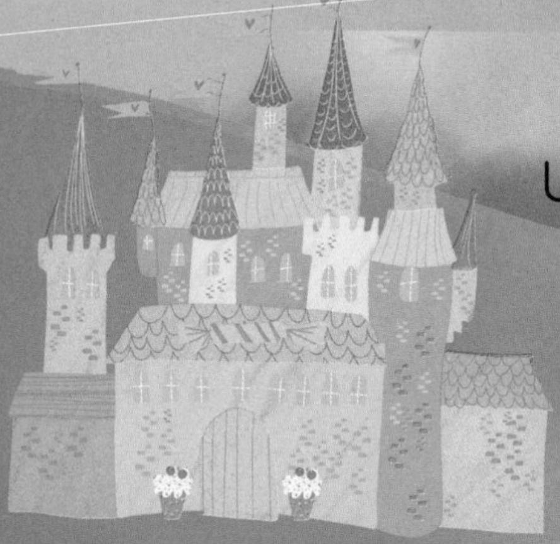

$90 \div 6$

	10	
6		

$91 \div 7$

	10	
7		

$84 \div 4$

	10	
4		

$104 \div 8$

	10	
8		

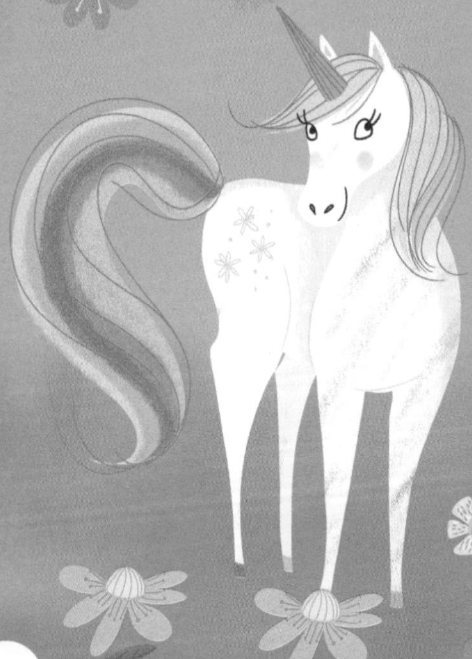

$64 \div 4$

	10	
4		

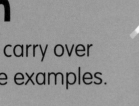

Short Division

Now try this. Divide the tens first, and carry over any remaining tens to the units, like the examples.

$$6 \overline{)7^18} \quad 13$$

$$3 \overline{)7^15} \quad 25$$

$$3 \overline{)81}$$

$$5 \overline{)95}$$

$$6 \overline{)84}$$

$$2 \overline{)76}$$

$$3 \overline{)84}$$

$$4 \overline{)84}$$

$$7 \overline{)98}$$

$$3 \overline{)63}$$

$$6 \overline{)96}$$

$$4 \overline{)64}$$

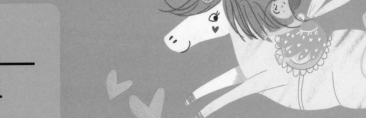

Bake Me a Cookie

Bella sells jars containing 11 of her delicious cookies.
Work out these calculations for her.

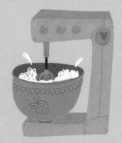

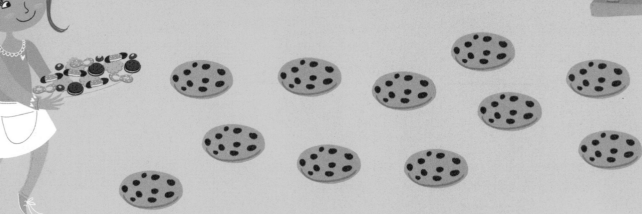

She has orders for nine jars.
How many cookies should she bake?

On Wednesday she bakes 100 cookies.
How many jars will that fill?

How many will be left over?

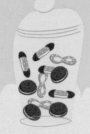

The ingredients for each jar cost 1.21.
How much does each cookie cost?

She plans to send 2 jars to the school,
3 jars to the care home, and 1 jar to the fire station.
How many cookies should she bake?

Present Practice

Match each of the unicorns to the correct present by working out the answers. Use short division.

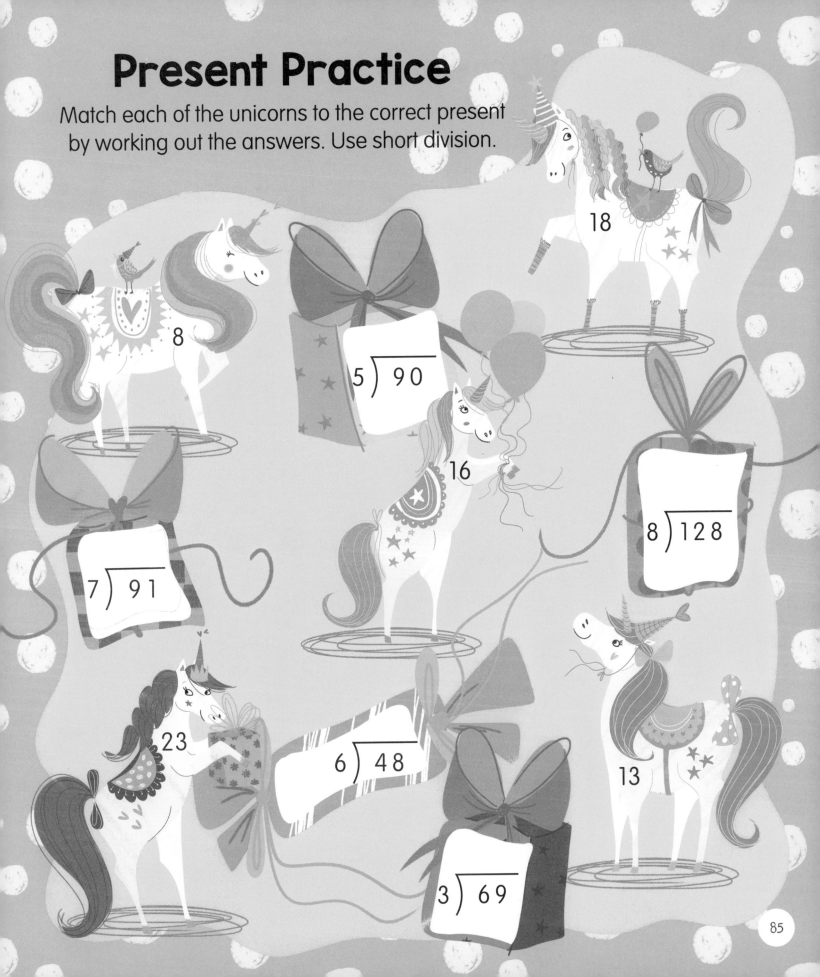

18

8

$5\overline{)90}$

16

$8\overline{)128}$

$7\overline{)91}$

23

$6\overline{)48}$

13

$3\overline{)69}$

Homework Help

Willow and Wanda have done their homework. Each of them has made some mistakes; can you find them?

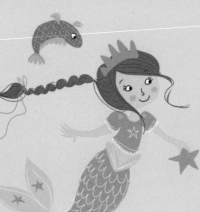
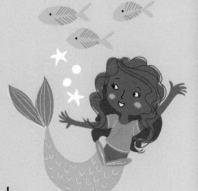

Willow	Wanda

26 x 7

x	2	6
7	14	42

56

x	20	6
7	140	42

182

123 x 6

x	100	20	3
6	600	120	18

738

```
  Th H T U
     1 2 3
         6
   -------
     8 3 8
   -------
```

28 x 8

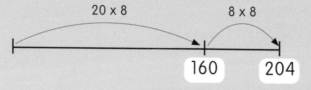

160   204

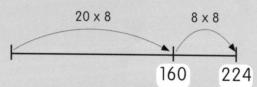

160   224

96 ÷ 4

```
      24
   4 ) 9 6
```

```
      21
   4 ) 9 6
```

100 x 10

10000

1000

Answers

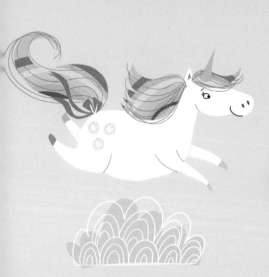

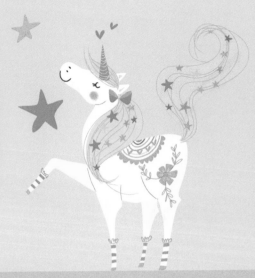

4 Sequences of Ten

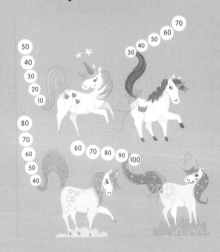

50
40
30
20
10

80
70
60
50
40

30 40 50 60 70

60 70 80 90 100

5 Sweet Treats

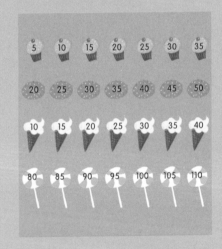

| 5 | 10 | 15 | 20 | 25 | 30 | 35 |

| 20 | 25 | 30 | 35 | 40 | 45 | 50 |

| 10 | 15 | 20 | 25 | 30 | 35 | 40 |

| 80 | 85 | 90 | 95 | 100 | 105 | 110 |

6 Under the Sea

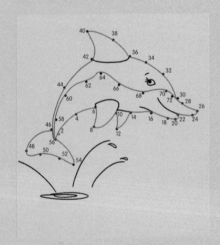

7 Totally Tropical

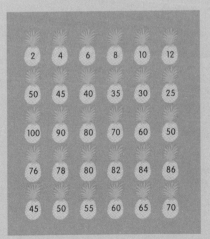

2	4	6	8	10	12
50	45	40	35	30	25
100	90	80	70	60	50
76	78	80	82	84	86
45	50	55	60	65	70

8 Again and Again

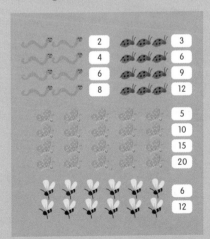

	2		3
	4		6
	6		9
	8		12

| 5 |
| 10 |
| 15 |
| 20 |

| 6 |
| 12 |

9 Now Multiply

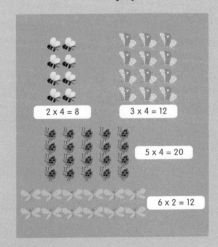

2 x 4 = 8   3 x 4 = 12

5 x 4 = 20

6 x 2 = 12

87

10 Food for Thought

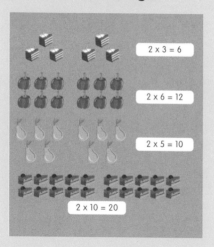

2 x 3 = 6

2 x 6 = 12

2 x 5 = 10

2 x 10 = 20

11 More Food for Thought

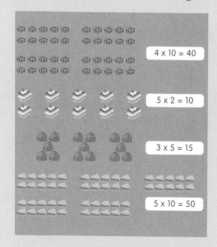

4 x 10 = 40

5 x 2 = 10

3 x 5 = 15

5 x 10 = 50

12 All Square

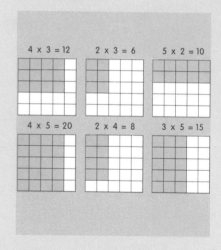

4 x 3 = 12   2 x 3 = 6   5 x 2 = 10

4 x 5 = 20   2 x 4 = 8   3 x 5 = 15

13 Castle Array

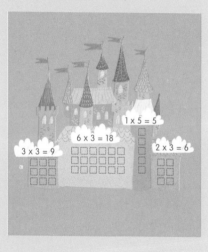

1 x 5 = 5

6 x 3 = 18

3 x 3 = 9

2 x 3 = 6

14 Double Trouble

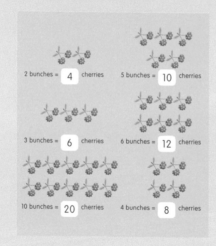

2 bunches = 4 cherries   5 bunches = 10 cherries

3 bunches = 6 cherries   6 bunches = 12 cherries

10 bunches = 20 cherries   4 bunches = 8 cherries

15 Sharing is Caring

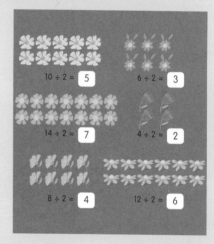

10 ÷ 2 = 5   6 ÷ 2 = 3

14 ÷ 2 = 7   4 ÷ 2 = 2

8 ÷ 2 = 4   12 ÷ 2 = 6

16 Ribbit!

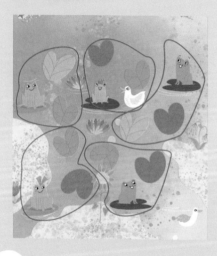

17 Spotted

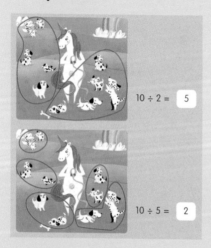

10 ÷ 2 = 5

10 ÷ 5 = 2

18 Undersea Treasures

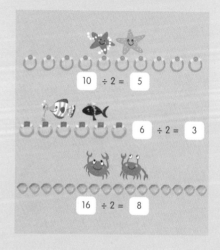

10 ÷ 2 = 5

6 ÷ 2 = 3

16 ÷ 2 = 8

19 Merpeople Treasure

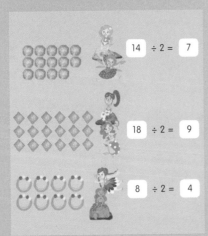

$14 \div 2 = 7$

$18 \div 2 = 9$

$8 \div 2 = 4$

20 Lighting the Night

$1 \times 2 = 2$	$7 \times 2 = 14$
$2 \times 2 = 4$	$8 \times 2 = 16$
$3 \times 2 = 6$	$9 \times 2 = 18$
$4 \times 2 = 8$	$10 \times 2 = 20$
$5 \times 2 = 10$	$11 \times 2 = 22$
$6 \times 2 = 12$	$12 \times 2 = 24$

21 Heading for Home

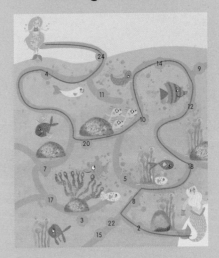

22 Flying High

$1 \times 10 = 10$	$7 \times 10 = 70$
$2 \times 10 = 20$	$8 \times 10 = 80$
$3 \times 10 = 30$	$9 \times 10 = 90$
$4 \times 10 = 40$	$10 \times 10 = 100$
$5 \times 10 = 50$	$11 \times 10 = 110$
$6 \times 10 = 60$	$12 \times 10 = 120$

23 In the Circle

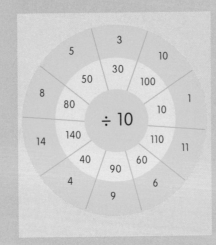

$\div 10$

24 Fairy Fives

$1 \times 5 = 5$	$7 \times 5 = 35$
$2 \times 5 = 10$	$8 \times 5 = 40$
$3 \times 5 = 15$	$9 \times 5 = 45$
$4 \times 5 = 20$	$10 \times 5 = 50$
$5 \times 5 = 25$	$11 \times 5 = 55$
$6 \times 5 = 30$	$12 \times 5 = 60$

25 Give Me Five

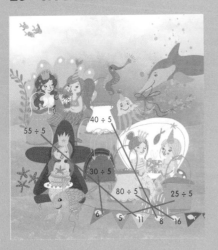

$55 \div 5$

$40 \div 5$

$30 \div 5$

$80 \div 5$

$25 \div 5$

26 In the Kitchen

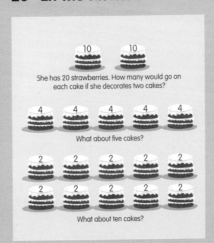

She has 20 strawberries. How many would go on each cake if she decorates two cakes?

What about five cakes?

What about ten cakes?

27 Squirrel Away

How many will there be if she divides them between 2 hiding places?

$20 \div 2 = 10$

How many will there be if she divides them between 5 hiding places?

$20 \div 5 = 4$

How many will there be if she divides them between 10 hiding places?

$20 \div 10 = 2$

28 Thirsty Work

1 x 3 = 3   7 x 3 = 21
2 x 3 = 6   8 x 3 = 24
3 x 3 = 9   9 x 3 = 27
4 x 3 = 12   10 x 3 = 30
5 x 3 = 15   11 x 3 = 33
6 x 3 = 18   12 x 3 = 36

29 Threes in the Sea

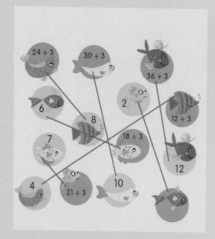

30 Wish on a Star

1 x 4 = 4   7 x 4 = 28
2 x 4 = 8   8 x 4 = 32
3 x 4 = 12   9 x 4 = 36
4 x 4 = 16   10 x 4 = 40
5 x 4 = 20   11 x 4 = 44
6 x 4 = 24   12 x 4 = 48

31 Hidden Treasure

8 goblets	2	2	2	2
12 ruby rings	3	3	3	3
4 diamonds	1	1	1	1
16 bracelets	4	4	4	4
20 brooches	5	5	5	5
24 coins	6	6	6	6

32 Whatever the Weather

1 x 6 = 6   7 x 6 = 42
2 x 6 = 12   8 x 6 = 48
3 x 6 = 18   9 x 6 = 54
4 x 6 = 24   10 x 6 = 60
5 x 6 = 30   11 x 6 = 66
6 x 6 = 36   12 x 6 = 72

33 Factors With Six

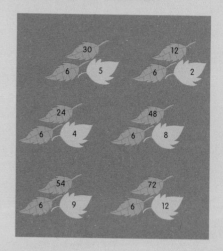

30   6   5   12   6   2
24   6   4   48   6   8
54   6   9   72   6   12

34 Visiting Friends

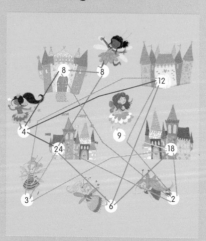

35 In the Kitchen

Share them between six friends.   4

Share them between four friends.   6

Share them between three friends.   8

They eat two cookies each. Now how many will there be shared between four friends?   5

36 Wonderful Water

1 x 7 = 7   7 x 7 = 49
2 x 7 = 14   8 x 7 = 56
3 x 7 = 21   9 x 7 = 63
4 x 7 = 28   10 x 7 = 70
5 x 7 = 35   11 x 7 = 77
6 x 7 = 42   12 x 7 = 84

37 Seahorse Sevens

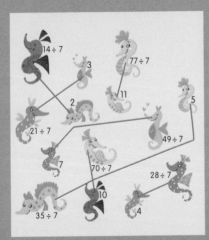

38 Fairy Rings

1 x 8 = 8	7 x 8 = 56
2 x 8 = 16	8 x 8 = 64
3 x 8 = 24	9 x 8 = 72
4 x 8 = 32	10 x 8 = 80
5 x 8 = 40	11 x 8 = 88
6 x 8 = 48	12 x 8 = 96

39 Eight Times Table

80	40	24		10	5	3
56	32	88	÷ 8 =	7	4	11
16	72	8		2	9	1
48	64	96		6	8	12

8	72	56		1	9	7
24	40	80		3	5	10
32	16	64	÷ 8 =	4	2	8
96	48	88		12	6	11

40 Beautiful Bunches

1 x 9 = 9	7 x 9 = 63
2 x 9 = 18	8 x 9 = 72
3 x 9 = 27	9 x 9 = 81
4 x 9 = 36	10 x 9 = 90
5 x 9 = 45	11 x 9 = 99
6 x 9 = 54	12 x 9 = 108

41 Sound Asleep

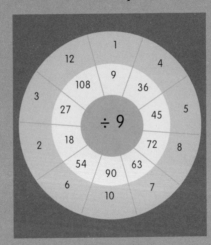

42 Days in the Sun

1 x 11 = 11	7 x 11 = 77
2 x 11 = 22	8 x 11 = 88
3 x 11 = 33	9 x 11 = 99
4 x 11 = 44	10 x 11 = 110
5 x 11 = 55	11 x 11 = 121
6 x 11 = 66	12 x 11 = 132

43 Spot It!

66	132	77		66	88	22
44	22	(101)	÷ 11	110	77	132
99	11	33		(111)	11	121
121	88	55		33	44	99

44	77	55		(140)	88	33
11	121	88	÷ 11	132	99	11
132	22	110		66	44	22
(91)	33	99		121	55	110

44 Happy Times

1 x 12 = 12	7 x 12 = 84
2 x 12 = 24	8 x 12 = 96
3 x 12 = 36	9 x 12 = 108
4 x 12 = 48	10 x 12 = 120
5 x 12 = 60	11 x 12 = 132
6 x 12 = 72	12 x 12 = 144

45 Sweet Music

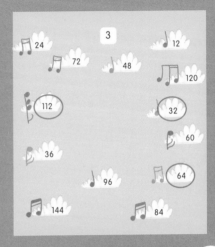

46 A Tough One

1	2	3	4	5	6	7	8	9	10	11	12
2	4	6	8	10	12	14	16	18	20	22	24
3	6	9	12	15	18	21	24	27	30	33	36
4	8	12	16	20	24	28	32	36	40	44	48
5	10	15	20	25	30	35	40	45	50	55	60
6	12	18	24	30	36	42	48	54	60	66	72
7	14	21	28	35	42	49	56	63	70	77	84
8	16	24	32	40	48	56	64	72	80	88	96
9	18	27	36	45	54	63	72	81	90	99	108
10	20	30	40	50	60	70	80	90	100	110	120
11	22	33	44	55	66	77	88	99	110	121	132
12	24	36	48	60	72	84	96	108	120	132	144

47 Fairy Factors

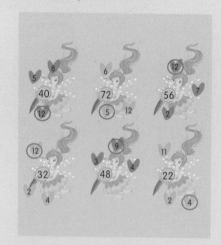

48 Daisy Chains

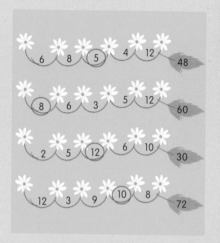

49 Feeling Crabby

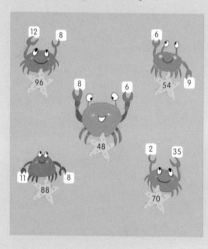

50 Octo-Puzzle

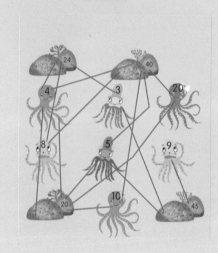

51 A Thing of Beauty

How many will there be on each bush, if an equal number land on each of six bushes? **4**

How many will there be on each bush, if an equal number land on each of four bushes? **6**

How many will there be on each bush, if an equal number land on each of three bushes? **8**

Six more butterflies appear! Now how many are there if they land in equal numbers on six bushes? **5**

52 Prime Numbers

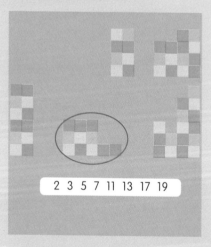

2 3 5 7 11 13 17 19

53 In the Air

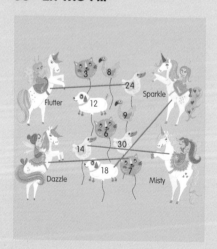

54 Scaling Solutions

You get an order for 10 chocolate and three times that number of vanilla. How many cakes in total do you have to make? **40**

You make 100 rainbow cakes and half that amount of lemon cakes. How many lemon cakes is that? **50**

If you can bake 24 cakes in an hour, how many can you bake in 3 hours? **72**

Chocolate cakes sell three times as many as strawberry. You sell 15 strawberry cupcakes in an hour. How many chocolate do you sell in the same time? **45**

You decorate each vanilla cake with two cherries. How many cherries will 80 cakes need? **160**

55 Bird Watching

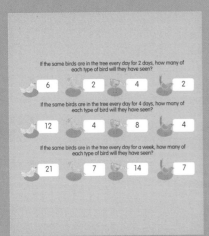

If the same birds are in the tree every day for 2 days, how many of each type of bird will they have seen?

| 6 | 2 | 4 | 2 |

If the same birds are in the tree every day for 4 days, how many of each type of bird will they have seen?

| 12 | 4 | 8 | 4 |

If the same birds are in the tree every day for a week, how many of each type of bird will they have seen?

| 21 | 7 | 14 | 7 |

56 Festive Fun

$8 \times 5 = 40$ $32 \div 4 = 8$

$11 \times 9 = 99$ $36 \div 9 = 4$

$9 \times 2 = 18$ $60 \div 12 = 5$

$7 \times 7 = 49$ $16 \div 8 = 2$

$6 \times 4 = 24$ $55 \div 11 = 5$

57 Hide and Seek

$2 \times 7 = 14$ $24 \div 3 = 8$

$8 \times 8 = 64$ $7 \times 5 = 35$

$54 \div 9 = 6$ $63 \div 9 = 7$

$28 \div 4 = 7$ $12 \div 2 = 6$

$49 \div 7 = 7$ $6 \times 3 = 18$

58 Whoops!

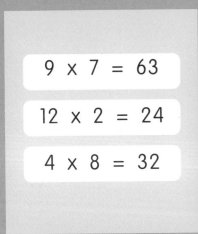

$9 \times 7 = 63$

$12 \times 2 = 24$

$4 \times 8 = 32$

59 Coral Calculations

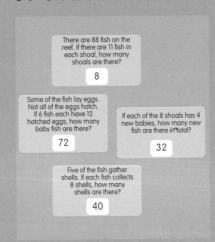

There are 88 fish on the reef. If there are 11 fish in each shoal, how many shoals are there?

8

Some of the fish lay eggs. Not all of the eggs hatch. If 6 fish each have 12 hatched eggs, how many baby fish are there?

72

If each of the 8 shoals has 4 new babies, how many new fish are there in total?

32

Five of the fish gather shells. If each fish collects 8 shells, how many shells are there?

40

60 One to One

$4 \times 1 = 4$ $8 \times 1 = 8$

$10 \times 1 = 10$ $20 \times 1 = 20$

$5 \times 1 = 5$ $50 \times 1 = 50$

$4 \div 1 = 4$ $20 \div 1 = 20$

$8 \div 1 = 8$ $15 \div 1 = 15$

$5 \div 1 = 5$ $50 \div 1 = 50$

61 Zero Zone

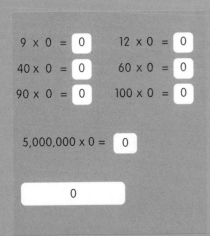

$9 \times 0 = 0$ $12 \times 0 = 0$

$40 \times 0 = 0$ $60 \times 0 = 0$

$90 \times 0 = 0$ $100 \times 0 = 0$

$5,000,000 \times 0 = 0$

0

62 Cutie Pies

x 10	Hundreds	Tens	Units
2	0	2	0
20	2	0	0
6	0	6	0
11	1	1	0
16	1	6	0
4	0	4	0
18	1	8	0
33	3	3	0
88	8	8	0

63 Mathematical Mirrors

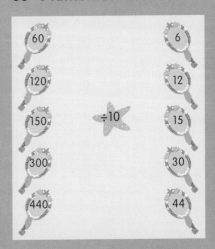

60	6
120	12
150	÷10	15
300	30
440	44

64 The Hundreds Table

x 100	Thousands	Hundreds	Tens	Units
1	0	1	0	0
20	2	0	0	0
5	0	5	0	0
18	1	8	0	0
33	3	3	0	0
9	0	9	0	0
12	1	2	0	0
66	6	6	0	0
88	8	8	0	0

65 Pool Party

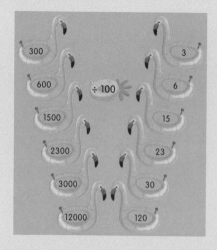

÷ 100

300, 3, 600, 6, 1500, 15, 2300, 23, 3000, 30, 12000, 120

66 Superstars

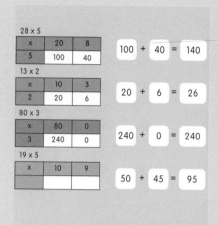

28 x 5

x	20	8
5	100	40

100 + 40 = 140

13 x 2

x	10	3
2	20	6

20 + 6 = 26

80 x 3

x	80	0
3	240	0

240 + 0 = 240

19 x 5

x	10	9

50 + 45 = 95

67 Tough Task

14 x 4

x	10	4
4	40	16

56

27 x 5

x	20	7
5	100	35

135

19 x 6

x	10	9
6	60	54

114

43 x 4

x	40	3
4	160	12

172

38 x 8

x	30	8
8	240	64

304

68 Logic Task

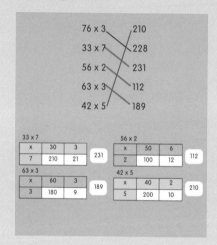

76 x 3 — 210
33 x 7 — 228
56 x 2 — 231
63 x 3 — 112
42 x 5 — 189

33 x 7

x	30	3
7	210	21

231

56 x 2

x	50	6
2	100	12

112

63 x 3

x	60	3
3	180	9

189

42 x 5

x	40	2
5	200	10

210

69 Taking Flight

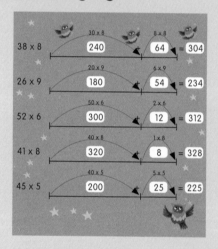

38 x 8: 30 x 8 = 240, 8 x 8 = 64, = 304
26 x 9: 20 x 9 = 180, 6 x 9 = 54, = 234
52 x 6: 50 x 6 = 300, 2 x 6 = 12, = 312
41 x 8: 40 x 8 = 320, 1 x 8 = 8, = 328
45 x 5: 40 x 5 = 200, 5 x 5 = 25, = 225

70 Something New

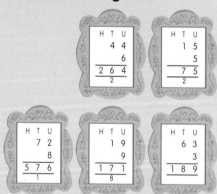

```
 H T U
   4 4
     6
 -----
 2 6 4
   2
```

```
 H T U
   1 5
     5
 -----
   7 5
   2
```

```
 H T U
   7 2
     8
 -----
 5 7 6
   1
```

```
 H T U
   1 9
     9
 -----
 1 7 1
   8
```

```
 H T U
   6 3
     3
 -----
 1 8 9
```

71 The Tea Room

	Pots of tea	Total cups (seven per pot)
Monday	12	84
Tuesday	16	112
Wednesday	27	189
Thursday	15	105
Friday	34	238
Saturday	39	273
Sunday	29	203

72 You Can Do It!

154 x 3

x	100	50	4
3	300	150	12

462

128 x 4

x	100	20	8
4	400	80	32

512

316 x 5

x	300	10	6
5	1500	50	30

1580

247 x 2

x	200	40	7
2	400	80	14

494

565 x 3

x	500	60	5
3	1500	180	15

1695

73 Do It Again!

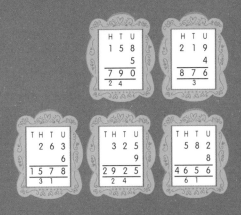

H T U
1 5 8
5
7 9 0
2 4

H T U
2 1 9
4
8 7 6
3

TH T U
2 6 3
6
1 5 7 8
3 1

TH T U
3 2 5
9
2 9 2 5
2 4

TH T U
5 8 2
8
4 6 5 6
6 1

74 Double Check

19 x 6	114
28 x 4	112
35 x 9	315
14 x 8	112
44 x 7	308

75 Check Again!

652 x 3	1956
271 x 6	1626
107 x 5	535
348 x 2	696
427 x 7	2989

76 Fairy Facts

22	x	4	=	88
4	x	22	=	88
88	÷	4	=	22
88	÷	22	=	4

33	x	3	=	99
3	x	33	=	99
99	÷	3	=	33
99	÷	33	=	3

16	x	4	=	64
4	x	16	=	64
64	÷	4	=	16
64	÷	16	=	4

77 Work It Out

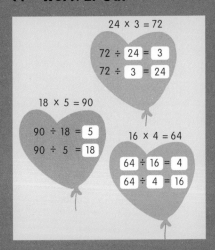

24 x 3 = 72

72 ÷ 24 = 3
72 ÷ 3 = 24

18 x 5 = 90

90 ÷ 18 = 5
90 ÷ 5 = 18

16 x 4 = 64

64 ÷ 16 = 4
64 ÷ 4 = 16

78 Festive Fun

2 x 6 = 12 12 ÷ 6 = 2	0
5 x 3 = 15 6 x 2 is 12 so 15 ÷ 6 = 2 with 3 left over	3
6 x 8 = 48 48 ÷ 6 = 8	0
2 x 12 = 24 24 ÷ 6 = 4	0
1 x 15 = 15 6 x 2 is 12 so 15 ÷ 6 = 2 with 3 left over	3
4 x 5 = 20 6 x 3 is 18 so 20 ÷ 6 = 3 with 2 left over	2

79 Delicious!

9	7
4	3
3	

80 Dividing Made Easy

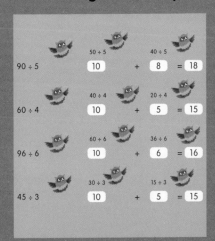

90 ÷ 5	50 ÷ 5	40 ÷ 5	
	10 +	8	= 18

60 ÷ 4	40 ÷ 4	20 ÷ 4	
	10 +	5	= 15

96 ÷ 6	60 ÷ 6	36 ÷ 6	
	10 +	6	= 16

45 ÷ 3	30 ÷ 3	15 ÷ 3	
	10 +	5	= 15

81 Dividing Bigger Numbers

38 ÷ 2

	10	9
2	20	18

10 + 9 = 19

96 ÷ 6

	10	6
6	60	36

10 + 6 = 16

57 ÷ 3

	10	9
3	30	27

10 + 9 = 19

90 ÷ 6

	10	5
6	60	30

15

91 ÷ 7

	10	3
7	70	21

13

84 ÷ 4

	10	11
4	40	44

21

104 ÷ 8

	10	3
8	80	24

13

64 ÷ 4

	10	6
4	40	24

16

83 Short Division

$$3\overline{)8^21} = 27$$

$$5\overline{)9^45} = 19 \qquad 6\overline{)8^24} = 14 \qquad 2\overline{)7^16} = 38$$

$$3\overline{)8^24} = 28 \qquad 4\overline{)84} = 21 \qquad 7\overline{)9^28} = 14$$

$$3\overline{)63} = 21 \qquad 6\overline{)9^36} = 16$$

$$4\overline{)6^24} = 16$$

84 Bake me a Cookie

99

9

1

0.11

66

85 Present Practice

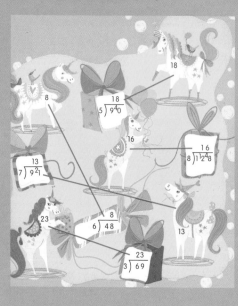

$$5\overline{)9^40} = 18$$
$$8\overline{)1^12^48} = 16$$
$$7\overline{)9^21} = 13$$
$$6\overline{)48} = 8$$
$$3\overline{)69} = 23$$

18, 16, 13, 23, 8

86 Homework Help

26 x 7

x	(2)	6
7	14	42

56

123 x 6

Th H T U
```
    1 2 3
        6
  (8) 3 8
```

28 x 8

20 x 8 → 160   8 x 8 → (204)

96 ÷ 4

$$4\overline{)9^16} = 21$$

100 x 10

1000(0)